RECIPES 4
RAW FOOD

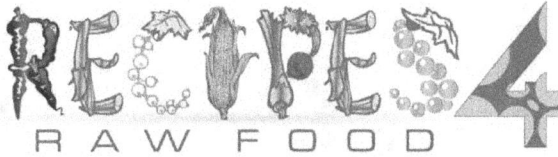

80 Awesome Raw Food Recipes You Can't Live Without

A COLLECTION OF 80 GREAT RAW RECIPES THAT ARE EASY, FUN, AND HEALTHY FOR EVERY MEAL!

BY KATHY TENNEFOSS

MEMBER OF THE RAW FOODS ASSOCIATION

RECIPES 4 RAW FOOD

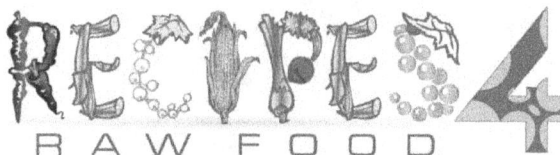

80 Awesome Raw Food Recipes You Can't Live Without

Sunny Cabana Publishing, L.L.C.

New Orleans, LA 70115

www.sunnycabanapublishing.com

By Kathy Tennefoss

All Rights Reserved © 2011 by Kathy Tennefoss

Published by Kathleen Tennefoss
Printed in the United States of America
Author: Kathy Tennefoss
Editor: Shawn M Tennefoss
13-digit ISBN: 1936874008
10-digit ISBN: 9781936874002
FIRST EDITION
Library of Congress Cataloging-in-Publication Data has been applied for

THIS BOOK IS DEDICATED TO MY DAD
JAMES KELLEY FOR PUSHING ME IN THE
RIGHT DIRECTION REGARDING HEALTHY
EATING, LIVING A HEALTHY ACTIVE LIFE,
AND TO MY LOVING HUSBAND SHAWN
TENNEFOSS FOR SUFFERING THROUGH MY
COMPUTER DIFFICULTIES AND TAKING THE
TIME TO SHOW ME HOW TO ORCHESTRATE
THIS BOOK ALONG WITH SHARING HIS
LIFE AND JOURNEY WITH ME.

COVER DESIGN:
KATHY & SHAWN TENNEFOSS

FIRST EDITION, 2011

ACKNOWLEDGEMENTS:

THANKS TO EVERYONE WHO ENCOURAGED
AND INSPIRED ME AND GAVE ME EXCELLENT
INPUT AND FEEDBACK IN THE RAW FOOD
INDUSTRY, INCLUDING ONE OF MY MANY
SISTERS HEATHER MCNERNEY, MY
HUSBAND SHAWN M TENNEFOSS, MY DAD
JAMES KELLEY, AND MELISSA HERNANDEZ
AND HER WONDERFUL FAMILY! WITHOUT
EVERYONE'S INPUT I WOULD NOT HAVE

FINISHED THIS BOOK OR STARTED OTHER
RAW FOOD RECIPE BOOKS. I AM EXTREMELY
GRATEFUL TO EVERYONE.

IF YOU HAVE ANY SUGGESTIONS,
COMMENTS, OR CORRECTIONS PLEASE SEND
ME AN EMAIL TO
RECIPES4RAWFOOD@YAHOO.COM.

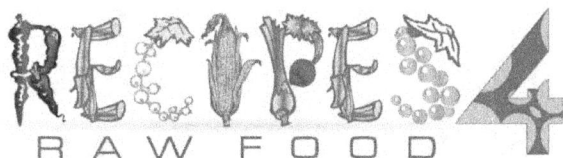

RECIPES4
RAW FOOD

DISCLAIMER:
THE RESPONSIBILITY FOR ANY ADVERSE
DETOXIFICATION EFFECTS RESULTING
FROM USING THESE RECIPES DESCRIBED
LIES NOT WITH THE AUTHOR OR
DISTRIBUTORS OF THIS BOOK. THIS BOOK
IS NOT INTENDED FOR MEDICAL ADVICE
JUST AS SUGGESTION.
PLEASE ENJOY THESE RECIPES WITH YOUR
FRIENDS AND FAMILY.

TABLE OF CONTENTS

INTRO

I HAVE PUT TOGETHER SOME GREAT RAW RECIPES THAT ARE EASY FOR YOU AND YOUR FAMILY TO MAKE. MAKING HEALTHY MEALS TOGETHER HELPS TO SOLIDIFY YOUR FAMILY VALUES AND BRING YOUR FAMILY CLOSER.

IN THIS RAW FOOD BOOK I HAVE GONE THROUGH ONLY SOME OF MY FAVORITE RAW RECIPES THAT I FOUND ARE THE EASIEST TO MAKE WHEN YOU ARE SHORT ON TIME. EVERYONE IS BUSY BUT YOU STILL SHOULD MAKE THE TIME TO EAT A HEALTHY MEAL. IT'S ALSO ABOUT PUTTING FUN INTO YOUR MEALS BY INVOLVING THE WHOLE FAMILY AND HAVE THEM HELP AND GIVE THEIR INPUT SO THAT THEY FEEL LIKE THEY ARE CONTRIBUTING TO THEIR OWN HEALTH BECAUSE WHEN YOUR CHILDREN GET OLDER THEY WILL REMEMBER THIS AND PASS THE HEALTHY LIVING ON TO THEIR CHILDREN. I KNOW THIS FROM EXPERIENCE. I

HAD A FATHER WHO ATE HEALTHY MOSTLY VEGETARIAN MEALS AND BIKED AND A MOTHER WHO ATE ONLY JUNK FOOD AND DID NOT EXERCISE WHATSOEVER. IT WAS A BATTLE AT OUR HOUSE OF WHAT TO EAT. I NEVER KNEW WHO TO GO WITH AS A CHILD BUT AT LEAST I HAD THE OPTION WHEN I GOT OLDER AND THAT IS WHY I FEEL SO COMPELLED TO TELL OTHERS ABOUT HEALTHY EATING.

I DIDN'T REALIZE UNTIL I GOT OLDER HOW MY DAD INFLUENCED ME AND MY FOOD CHOICES. MY MOTHER WAS ALWAYS SICK AND DID NOT TAKE CARE OF HERSELF VERY WELL AND THAT WAS TO HER DETRIMENT. I VOWED TO MYSELF AND MY FAMILY THAT I WOULD TRY MY HARDEST TO SEEK OUT THE BEST QUALITY FOOD BY PURCHASING ORGANIC PRODUCE AND BY PREPARING THE FOOD AS TO NOT LOSE ITS NUTRITIONAL VALUE AND I HAVE STUCK TO THAT PROMISE FOR OVER 20 YEARS. I FEEL THAT THIS HAS HELPED ME AND MY

FAMILY IMMENSELY AND I WANT TO PASS THE BENEFITS ON TO OTHERS SO THAT THEY TOO WILL FEEL THAT THEY ARE CONTRIBUTING TO A BETTER WAY OF LIFE!

PLEASE TRY ALL OF MY RECIPES AND PUT YOUR BEST FOOT FORWARD IN THE FIGHT FOR OBESITY, DIABETES, HEART DISEASE, CANCER, AND A SLEW OF OTHER AILMENTS THAT ARE FROM NOT EATING A HEALTHY DIET. ALSO REMEMBER THAT LIFE SHOULD BE FUN AND THAT EATING HEALTHY DOESN'T MEAN THAT YOU HAVE TO BE STRICT EVERY SINGLE DAY. IT'S THE SMALL EFFORTS THAT YOU PUT FORTH EVERYDAY THAT MAKE A DIFFERENCE IN THE LONG RUN! PEOPLE WILL START TO NOTICE YOUR HEALTHY GLOW AND HOW YOUNG YOU LOOK AND START TO ASK YOU HOW, WHAT, AND WILL YOU SHOW ME. THIS IS WHEN YOU WILL FEEL LIKE YOU HAVE MADE A DIFFERENCE IN THE WORLD.

SOME HELPFUL TIPS AND USEFUL INFORMATION FOR YOUR RAW KITCHEN

RAW COCONUTS

THE SWEET AND SALTY OF RAW FOOD

TURN UP THE HEAT

ALOE VERA

RAW NUTS

RAW COCONUTS

IF YOU ARE NOT SURE ABOUT HOW TO USE A RAW YOUNG COCONUT HERE IS AN EASY SOLUTION FOR YOU.

YOUNG COCONUTS ARE NOT JUST A WONDERFUL DELICACY. THERE ARE SO MANY WAYS IN WHICH YOUNG COCONUTS DO WONDERS FOR OUR HEALTH LIKE LOWERING CHOLESTEROL, REDUCE THE RISK OF HEART DISEASE, AND HAS ANTI-INFLAMMATORY BENEFITS FOR THE BODY.

IN THE TROPICAL REGION IT IS CONSIDERED TO BE THE MOST IMPORTANT FRUIT, SIMPLY BECAUSE PEOPLE KNOW OF ITS MEDICINAL PROPERTIES AND ALSO BECAUSE OF ITS MINERAL RICH WATER, SUCH AS POTASSIUM, COPPER, IRON, CALCIUM, ASCORBIC ACID, AND B-COMPLEX VITAMINS. YOUNG COCONUTS ARE HIGHLY NUTRITIOUS IN NATURE AND HAVE MEDICATIVE QUALITIES, WHICH ARE VERY GOOD FOR YOUR HEART, LIVER AND KIDNEYS. IN FACT, THE LATEST RESEARCH REPORTS SUGGEST THAT APART FROM ITS

NUTRITIONAL FEATURES THE YOUNG COCONUTS ARE REPORTED TO REDUCE THE VIRAL LOAD OF HUMAN IMMUNO-DEFICIENCY VIRUS OR HIV.

IT'S ALSO KNOWN FOR ITS NATURAL ELECTROLYTE SOURCE. ALSO, IT IS BELIEVED THAT MANY PEOPLE LIVING IN THIRD WORLD COUNTRIES HAVE ACTUALLY BEEN SAVED BY THESE YOUNG COCONUTS. THE COCONUTS IN THEIR YOUNG AGE HAPPEN TO BE THE MOST HEALTH ENHANCING. NOT TO MENTION THE FACT THAT IT'S SIMILAR TO BLOOD PLASMA AND HAS BEEN USED IN EMERGENCY BLOOD TRANSFUSIONS.

THESE ARE JUST FEW OF THE BENEFITS OF YOUNG COCONUTS. NOW LET'S DISCUSS HOW TO OPEN AND EAT A YOUNG COCONUT AS MANY PEOPLE FIND THIS A TOUGH JOB TO DO:

THE BEST AND SIMPLEST WAY TO OPEN A COCONUT IS TO PUT THE COCONUT INSIDE A PLASTIC BAG, TIE ITS ENDS AND JUST SWING IT ON ANY FLAT, HARD SURFACE,

WHICH WOULD SHATTER THE YOUNG COCONUT INTO SHARDS. YOU CAN GET THE MEAT SIMPLY BY SEPARATING COCONUT MEAT FROM THE HUSK IN THIS FASHION. USE THE PLASTIC BAG TO RETAIN THE COCONUT WATER. NOW HOLD THE PLASTIC BAG SO THAT THE LIQUID SETTLES DOWN AT THE BOTTOM. YOU CAN NOW PUNCTURE A HOLE AND GET A GLASSFUL OF COCONUT JUICE. IT'S AS EASY AS 1, 2, 3. .

THE MEATS OF YOUNG COCONUT ARE QUITE SOFT AND CAN BE SCOOPED OUT WITH A SPOON OR A KNIFE. HOWEVER, THE SUGGESTED WAY IS TO USE A SMALL KNIFE WITH A FLEXIBLE BLADE, WHICH WOULD ALLOW IT TO FOLLOW THE CONTOUR OF THE SHELL WHILE UNDERCUTTING THE MEAT OUT OF THE SHELL.

THE YOUNG COCONUTS ARE GREAT CHOICE FOR THE SUMMERS AS THEY QUITE EASY TO PREPARE AND THEY ARE AVAILABLE AT MOST GROCERY STORE. YOUNG COCONUTS ARE A GREAT ENHANCER TO VARIOUS DRINKS, ESPECIALLY TROPICAL DRINKS, SMOOTHIES, PIES, AND DINNER DISHES AS

WELL. HUMID COUNTRIES RELY HEAVILY ON COCONUT-BASED FOODS.

THE SWEET AND SALTY OF RAW FOOD

FOR THE MOST PART YOU WILL EVENTUALLY USE SOME TYPE OF NATURAL SWEETENERS OR SALTY FLAVORING FOR YOUR RAW FOOD RECIPES. USING REFINED SUGARS ARE NOT BENEFICIAL TO THE BODY BECAUSE IT IMBALANCES THE BODY GIVES YOU AN ENERGY CRASH. COMPANIES HAVE BEEN TRYING TO MANUFACTURE SWEETENERS LIKE SACCHARINE AND ASPARTAME, WHICH HAVE REPORTS OF BEING TAKEN OFF THE MARKET FOR BEING TOXIC OR CAUSING CANCER, EITHER WAY IT DOESN'T SOUND THAT GREAT WHEN THERE ARE TONS OF NATURAL ALTERNATIVES OUT THERE IN THE SUPERMARKET.

MOST FOOD IN ITS RAW STATE IS FLAVORFUL WITHOUT IT BUT WHEN YOU ARE TRYING TO MAKE A RECIPE WITH COMBINED INGREDIENTS YOU WILL WANT TO USE EITHER CELTIC SALT, HIMALAYAN

SALT (THIS IS ONE OF MY FAVORITES DUE TO THE GREAT MINERAL CONTENT), OR OTHER FLAVORED SALTS THAT THEY HAVE ON THE MARKET. YOU CAN ALSO USE A PRODUCT CALLED BRAGGS LIQUID AMINO ACIDS (WHICH YOU CAN PURCHASE IN MOST HEALTH FOOD STORES) AS A SALT SUBSTITUTE. BRAGGS HAS MANY AMINO ACIDS AND ENZYMES THAT ARE NECESSARY FOR YOUR BODY TO FUNCTION PROPERLY AND IT IS NOT FERMENTED. YOU MAY ALSO USE A PRODUCT THAT IS CALLED NAMA SHOYU, WHICH IS A RAW FERMENTED SOY SAUCE FOR FLAVORING MANY DISHES.

AS FAR AS SWEET GOES ONE OF MY FAVORITE SWEETENERS TO USE IS AGAVE (CACTUS) NECTAR. I USE IT IN SMOOTHIES AND IN MY GREEN TEA BUT THERE ARE MANY OTHER WAYS TO SWEETEN YOUR RAW FOOD. YOU CAN USE DATE SUGAR (OR IF YOU DON'T HAVE DATE SUGAR YOU MAY USE JUST PLAIN DATES) WHICH, IS MADE OF GROUND UP DRIED DATES AND BY USING DATE SUGAR YOU HAVE ADDED FIBER TO YOUR RECIPE. WHAT A BONUS! YOU CAN

ALSO USE OTHER DRIED FRUITS THAT ARE GROUND UP IN A FOOD PROCESSOR. YOU WILL JUST HAVE TO EXPERIMENT TO SEE WHAT YOU LIKE BEST. RAW HONEY IS ALSO ANOTHER GREAT CHOICE. I HAVE USED THIS ON OCCASION. RAW HONEY IS HONEY THAT HAS NOT BEEN HEATED DURING THE EXTRACTION FROM THE HIVE. BY USING RAW HONEY YOU WILL ALSO HAVE THE BENEFITS OF ENZYMES, B-COMPLEX, AND MINERALS. ANOTHER ONE OF MY FAVORITES IS MAPLE SYRUP BECAUSE IT MIXES WELL IN LIQUIDS AND HAS TONS OF MINERALS AND A GREAT FLAVOR. TURBINADO SUGAR IS ANOTHER GOOD CHOICE THAT IS MADE FROM PARTIALLY REFINED RAW SUGAR WHICH CAN BE BETTER IF YOU WANT A SMOOTHER FINISH IN A DESSERT OR SMOOTHIE.

SO ALL IN ALL YOU WON'T REALLY MISS REFINED SUGAR OR TABLE SALT IF YOU JUST FOLLOW THE ABOVE CHOICES FOR YOUR NOW AND FUTURE RECIPES. PLUS YOU ARE ADDING MORE MINERALS, FIBER, ENZYMES, AND AMINO ACIDS TO YOUR DIET. SO LIFE CAN BE SWEETER AND FOR

YOU FOLKS THAT LIKE THINGS A LITTLE
SALTY TRY SOME NEW WAYS OF
FLAVORING YOUR MEALS.

TURN UP THE HEAT

THERE ARE MANY WAYS TO MAKE
YOUR RAW FOOD DISHES SPICY. HERE ARE
SOME OF MY FAVORITES: JALAPENOS,
HABANERA, SERRANO, BANANA, SCOTCH
BONNET, THAI PEPPERS, CHILIES, CAYENNE,
AND THE LIST GOES ON. THERE ARE OVER
20 VARIETALS OF PEPPERS AND NOT ALL OF
THEM ARE HOT BUT THEY DO ADD TONS OF
FLAVOR TO DISHES. YOU CAN USE THESE
IN THEIR RAW STATE OR DEHYDRATED
STATE FOR YOUR RECIPES. EITHER WAY
THEY WILL BOTH TASTE GREAT AND ADD
TONS OF FLAVOR, COLOR, AND HEALTH
BENEFITS. JUST REMEMBER THAT A LITTLE
GOES A LONG WAY! IT IS ALSO A GOOD
IDEA TO USE GLOVES WHEN CUTTING THEM
SO THAT YOU WON'T FORGET LATER AND
RUB YOUR EYES BECAUSE SOME OF THOSE
PEPPERS CAN BE VERY POTENT.

PEPPERS ARE BENEFICIAL TO THE BODY BECAUSE THEY HAVE VITAMIN A, C, AND K PLUS A GOOD AMOUNT OF FIBER. PEPPERS HELP PREVENT CELL DAMAGE, INFLAMMATION, ASTHMA, CANCER, DECREASE CHOLESTEROL, REDUCE ULCERS, SUPPORT IMMUNE FUNCTION AND CAN HELP WITH WEIGHT LOSS. THEY ONLY HAVE BETWEEN 10-20 CALORIES PER SERVING BUT THEY ADD SO MUCH FLAVOR AND SO MANY HEALTH BENEFITS TO YOUR BODY. HOW CAN YOU NOT LOVE THEM?

OTHER WAYS TO MAKE DISHES SPICY IS BY ADDING RAW GARLIC, GINGER, BASIL, HORSERADISH, ONIONS, OR SEAWEED. ALL OF THESE ARE SO BENEFICIAL FOR YOUR BODY AS WELL. GARLIC HAS BEEN KNOWN TO BE A POWERFUL NATURAL ANTIBIOTIC AND THERE HAVE BEEN STUDIES THAT HAVE SHOWN THAT GARLIC HAS REDUCED ONES CHOLESTEROL. GINGER IS ANOTHER GREAT ADDITION TO ANYONE'S DIET. GINGER HELPS WITH UPSET STOMACHS, NAUSEA, AND POOR DIGESTION. A COUPLE OF BENEFITS OF EATING BASIL ARE THAT IT HAS BEEN KNOWN TO HELP WITH

NAUSEA AND MOTION SICKNESS.
HORSERADISH HAS C AND B-COMPLEX
VITAMINS AND HAS BEEN USED TO TREAT
SUCH ILLNESSES AS TOOTHACHE, SCURVY,
COUGHS, ACHING JOINTS, AND DIABETES.
ONIONS HAVE BEEN USED TO TREAT
COLDS, COUGHS, AND ASTHMA. SEAWEED
OR SEA VEGETABLES HAVE SO MANY
BENEFITS FOR THE BODY AND THERE ARE
SO MANY DIFFERENT VARIETALS THAT I
CAN'T EVEN BEGIN TALK ABOUT THEM.
DULSE IS ONE OF MY FAVORITES AND
MAKES A GREAT ADDITION TO SALADS AND
RAW SOUPS.

YOU WILL FIND MANY HEALTH
BENEFITS AND HAVE A BLAST TRYING NEW
RECIPES WITH ALL OF THESE DIFFERENT
WAYS TO SPICE UP YOUR MEALS. THERE ARE
SO MANY BENEFITS TO MAKING YOUR
DISHES SPICY WHY WOULDN'T YOU SPICE
IT UP A BIT? SPICE IT UP FOR YOU AND
YOUR FAMILY'S HEALTH.

ALOE VERA

ALOE VERA WAS FIRST DISCOVERED AND CULTIVATED BY THE EGYPTIANS. ALOE VERA GROWS GREAT IN A TROPICAL ENVIRONMENT LIKE FLORIDA, HAWAII, OR THE CARIBBEAN.

I FEEL THAT ALOE VERA IS ONE OF THE MOST BENEFICIAL PLANTS AVAILABLE. ALOE VERA HAS VITAMIN C, A, E AND CALCIUM, CHROMIUM, SELENIUM, ZINC, MAGNESIUM, FIBER (HELPFUL WITH WEIGHT LOSS), ANTIOXIDANTS, LIGNIN'S, AMINO ACIDS, PLANT STEROLS (GOOD FOR HIGH CHOLESTEROL), AND POLYSACCHARIDES.

THE BENEFITS OF ALOE VERA ARE ASTONISHING. WHEN YOU DRINK ALOE VERA JUICE IT HELPS WITH LUBRICATING THE JOINTS, BRAIN, AND NERVOUS SYSTEM. IT IS ALSO VERY BENEFICIAL FOR THE SKIN BOTH INTERNALLY AND EXTERNALLY. IF YOU TEND TO WORK OUT A LOT OR EVEN A LITTLE THEN IT IS PROBABLY A GOOD IDEA TO ADD ALOE VERA

JUICE TO YOUR DIET SO THAT YOUR
JOINTS WILL LAST LONGER AND
FUNCTION BETTER.

ALOE VERA JUICE ALSO AIDS WITH
DIGESTION BY GIVING A CALMING EFFECT
TO THE COLON. IT HAS BEEN KNOWN TO
HELP WITH IBS AND ULCERS. I DRINK ALOE
VERA JUICE IF I HAVE AN UPSET STOMACH
AND IT HELPS RIGHT AWAY. NOW THE
TASTE IS SOMETHING THAT TOOK ME A
LITTLE WHILE TO GET USED TO BUT NOW
IT DOESN'T BOTHER ME AT ALL. PLUS YOU
CAN MIX IT IN WITH OTHER JUICES OR
SMOOTHIES TO HIDE THE FLAVOR.

ALOE VERA ALSO HAS BEEN SHOWN TO
HELP WITH BALANCING OUT THE BLOOD
SUGAR AND LESSENING THE SYMPTOMS OF
DIABETICS. MAYBE IF EVERYONE DRANK
ALOE VERA JUICE THEN WE WOULDN'T
HAVE AN EPIDEMIC OF DIABETES IN
AMERICA. IT SEEMS LIKE EVERYONE
KNOWS OF AT LEAST ONE PERSON IN
THEIR LIFE THAT HAS DIABETES. SO MAKE
IT YOUR QUEST TO HELP OTHERS BY

TELLING THEM THE HEALTH BENEFITS OF ALOE VERA JUICE.

IT IS ALSO VERY BENEFICIAL FOR THE SKIN BOTH INTERNALLY AND EXTERNALLY.

EXTERNALLY ALOE VERA IS GREAT FOR SO MANY THINGS LIKE POISON IVY OR OAK, RASHES, ACNE, ATHLETE'S FEET, BURNS, ECZEMA, INSECT STINGS OR BITES, JELLYFISH STINGS, STRETCH MARKS, SUNBURN, VARICOSE VEINS, AND ABRASIONS.

EVERYONE SHOULD HAVE A BOTTLE OF ORGANIC 100% ALOE VERA FOR TOPICAL TREATMENTS AND ALOE VERA JUICE TO TAKE CARE OF THE INSIDE OF YOUR BODY!

RAW NUTS

I ALSO WANTED TO INCLUDE SOME NFORMATION ON THE BENEFITS OF NUTS SINCE THEY ARE IN A LOT OF MY RECIPES AND ARE CONSIDERED A STAPLE IN THE RAW FOOD DIET.

ALMOST ALL OF THE DESSERTS HAVE
NUTS IN THEM AND I THINK THAT IT
WOULD BE GOOD FOR YOU TO KNOW
SOME OF THE BENEFITS OF THE NUTS
FOR YOU AND YOUR FAMILY.

NUTS ARE AN AMAZING FOOD. NUTS
ARE VERY BENEFICIAL FOR YOUR
HEALTH AND THEY TASTE GREAT TOO!
NUTS ARE HIGH IN CALORIES BUT THEY
ARE STILL VERY BENEFICIAL TO YOUR
BODY BECAUSE THEY ARE LOADED WITH
MONO SATURATED FATS, WHICH HELP
TO LOWER HEART DISEASE. MANY
NUTS ARE RICH IN OMEGA 3 FATTY
ACIDS. OMEGA 3 ESSENTIAL FATTY
ACIDS ARE GOOD FOR YOUR HEART AND
FOR YOUR ARTERIES. OMEGA 3
ESSENTIAL FATTY ACIDS ARE HELPFUL
FOR MAKING YOUR HEART RHYMES
MORE STABLE SO YOU CAN TRY TO
AVOID A HEART ATTACK. NUTS ALSO
HAVE L-ARGININE WHICH IS HELPFUL
TO YOUR HEART AND ARTERIES

BECAUSE IT MAKES YOUR ARTERIES MORE FLEXIBLE AND LEADS TO LESS BLOOD CLOTS. NUTS ALSO HAVE BEEN KNOWN TO HAVE PLANT STEROLS IN THEM WHICH HELP TO LOWER CHOLESTEROL.

IT IS BEST TO EAT NUTS RAW, SOAKED, OR SPROUTED BECAUSE THEY ARE CONSIDERED TO BE LIVE FOODS. LIVE FOODS ARE FOODS THAT HAVE NOT BEEN HEATED AT HIGH TEMPERATURES OR COOKED. HEATING NUTS TO ABOVE 118 DEGREES STARTS TO DESTROY BENEFICIAL ENZYMES. WHEN THESE ENZYMES ARE DESTROYED THE NUTS ARE UNABLE TO SPROUT SO THEY WOULD BE CONSIDERED NOT LIVE.

SOME OF THE BEST RAW NUTS ARE WALNUTS, CASHEWS, BRAZIL, MACADAMIA, ALMONDS, PECANS, AND FILBERTS. THEY ALSO MAKE GREAT MILKS WHEN PROCESSED CORRECTLY. ALMONDS ARE ONE OF MY FAVORITE

NUTS THEY ARE HIGH IN PROTEIN, VITAMIN E, MAGNESIUM, ZINC, POTASSIUM, AND IRON. ALMONDS ALSO HAVE THE HIGHEST AMOUNT OF CALCIUM OF ANY OTHER NUT SO THEY MAKE A GREAT SUBSTITUTE FOR DAIRY PRODUCTS FOR RAW FOODIST AND VEGANS. ALMONDS ALSO HAVE SOME OF THE HIGHEST FIBER CONTENT OF ANY OTHER NUT. CASHEWS ARE ANOTHER GOOD NUT BUT SHOULD BE REFRIGERATED ONCE THE PACKAGE IS OPENED BECAUSE THE SPOIL EASILY. CASHEWS ARE HIGH IN COPPER AND MAGNESIUM. CASHEWS ALSO HAVE ONE OF THE LOWEST FAT CONTENT OF ANY OTHER NUT. MACADAMIA NUTS ARE ALSO ONE OF MY FAVORITES. MACADAMIA NUTS ARE A HIGH ENERGY FOOD AND CONTAIN NO CHOLESTEROL. THE NATURAL OILS IN MACADAMIAS CONTAIN 78% MONOUNSATURATED FATS, THE HIGHEST OF ANY OIL INCLUDING OLIVE OIL. MACADAMIAS

CONTAIN TOCOPHEROLS AND TOCOTRIENOLS, WHICH ARE DERIVATIVES OF VITAMIN E, PHYTOSTEROLS SUCH AS SITOSTEROL AND ALSO SELENIUM. ONE OF THE BEST NUTS FOR YOUR HEALTH ARE WALNUTS. WALNUTS ARE ONE OF THE BEST SOURCES OF OMEGA 3 ESSENTIAL FATTY ACIDS AND THEY HAVE MORE ANTIOXIDANTS THAN MOST OTHER NUTS. BRAZIL NUTS ARE EXTREMELY NUTRIENT RICH AND HIGH IN ANTIOXIDANTS LIKE SELENIUM WHICH HELPS TO NEUTRALIZE FREE RADICALS. FILBERTS ARE ALSO VERY BENEFICIAL. IF YOU ADD FILBERTS TO YOUR SALADS OR SMOOTHIES THEN THEY HELP YOU TO ABSORB THE FAT SOLUBLE VITAMINS A, D, E, AND K. FILBERTS ARE ALSO GREAT FOR ANTI AGING PROPERTIES SUCH AS ALZHEIMER'S, STROKE, ARTHRITIS, WRINKLES, AND HEART DISEASE.

ALMOST ALL NUTS HAVE PHOTO NUTRIENTS WHICH ARE BIOLOGICALLY ACTIVE COMPONENTS THAT PROTECT OUR BODIES SYSTEMS. MANY NUTS ACT AS ANTIOXIDANTS, WHICH SCAVENGE THE FREE RADICALS THAT OXIDIZE BLOOD FATS. PHOTO NUTRIENTS OPERATE AS PART OF COMPLEX SYSTEMS THAT ARE ONLY PARTLY UNDERSTOOD.

NUTS ARE AN AMAZING FOOD! THEY ARE SO GOOD FOR YOU AND THEY TASTE GREAT AND CAN BE USED IN SO MANY RAW AND VEGAN RECIPES BUT JUST BE CAREFUL TO NOT OVER EAT THEM BECAUSE THEY ARE HIGH IN CALORIES.

20 Super Smoothies

POPEYE'S GREEN MACHINE

STRAWBERRY GREEN MACHINE

GREENELOUPE

WHAT THE KALE

MANGO MAMMA

ACAI SUPER CHARGER

PEACHES & GREEN

GREEN APPLE

GREEN KIWI

CUCUMBER MADNESS

CHOCOLATE HEAVEN

TROPICAL PAPAYA

SWEET CHERRY

GREEN TEA SMOOTHIE

BLUEBERRY GINGER SMOOTHIE

PEAR SMOOTHIE

GREEN NECTARINE

BLACKBERRY DREAM

MIXED GREEN BERRY

FIGLISIOUS

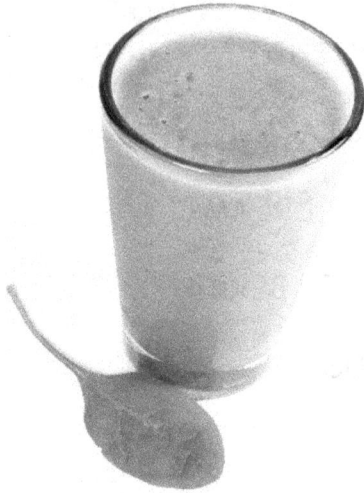

POPEYE'S GREEN MACHINE

1 CUP ALMOND MILK

2 CUPS SPINACH

$\frac{1}{4}$ CUP ALOE VERA JUICE

1 SCOOP RAW MEAL REPLACEMENT (I USE GARDEN OF LIFE)

1 CUP BLUEBERRIES

SPLASH OF LIME JUICE

1 CUP OF ICE

MIX THIS ALL IN A VITA MIXER OR
BLENDER AND SERVE. THIS MAKES TWO
SMALL GLASSES OR ONE LARGE GLASS.

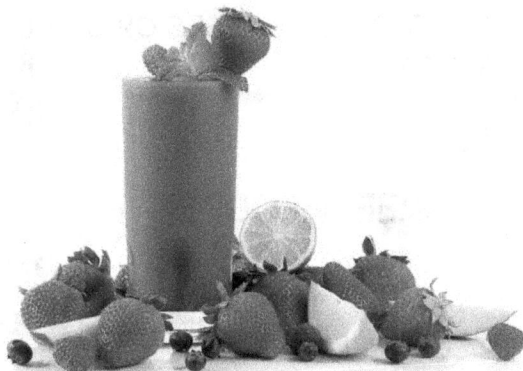

STRAWBERRY GREEN DREAM

1 CUP ALMOND MILK

1 CUP SPINACH

1 CUP CELERY

¼ ALOE VERA JUICE

1 SCOOP RAW MEAL REPLACEMENT

1 CUP STRAWBERRIES

$\frac{1}{4}$ CUP LIME JUICE

1 CUP OF ICE

MIX ALL THE INGREDIENTS IN A VITA MIXER AND A BLENDER AND SERVE. THIS MAKES TWO GLASSES OR ONE LARGE GLASS.

GREENELOUPE

2 CUPS CELERY

1 CUP ALMOND MILK

1 CUP CANTALOUPE

$\frac{1}{4}$ CUP LIME JUICE

1 SCOOP RAW MEAL REPLACEMENT

1 CUP OF ICE

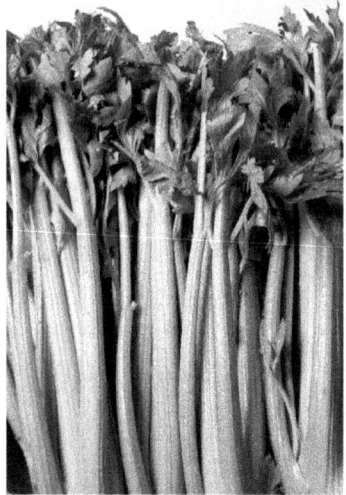

MIX ALL INGREDIENTS IN A VITA MIXER
OR BLENDER AND SERVE. THIS MAKES TWO
MEDIUM GLASSES.

WHAT THE KALE

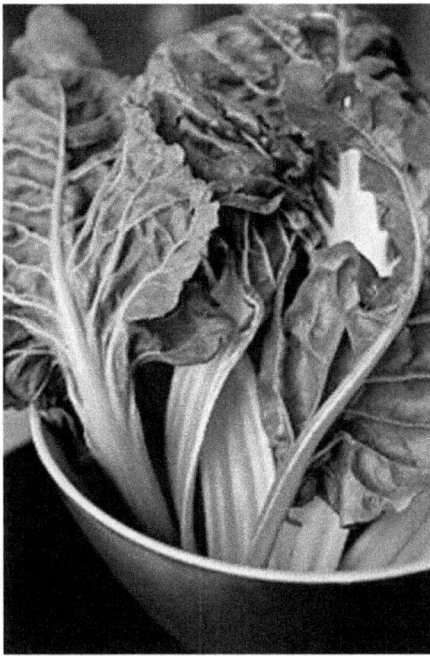

2 CUPS GREEN KALE

1 FROZEN BANANA (WHEN YOUR BANANAS
START TO GET TO RIPE ITS BEST TO PEEL
THEM AND SLICE THEM IN SMALLER PIECES

SO THAT YOU CAN USE THEM LATER IN SMOOTHIES)

1 CUP ALMOND MILK

5-7 MEDIUM STRAWBERRIES

1 CUP BLUEBERRIES

1 SCOOP RAW FOOD MEAL REPLACEMENT

1 CUP OF ICE

MIX INGREDIENTS IN A VITA MIXER OR BLENDER AND SERVE. THIS MAKES TWO MEDIUM GLASSES.

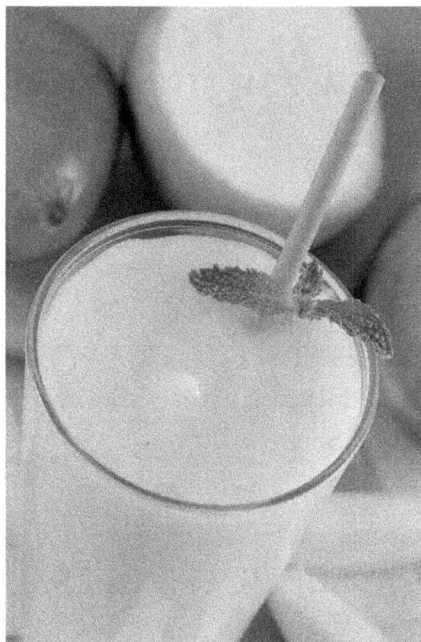

MANGO MAMMA

1 CUP FROZEN MANGOS (YOU CAN USE
FRESH IF YOU HAVE IT BUT THE
CONSISTENCY WILL BE A LITTLE THINNER)

2 CUPS OF CELERY

½ CUP ALMOND MILK

½ CUP ORANGE JUICE

½ FROZEN BANANA

1 SCOOP OF RAW MEAL REPLACEMENT

1 SEEDED DATE

1 TABLESPOON COCONUT OIL

1 CUP OF ICE

BLEND ALL INGREDIENTS IN A VITA MIXER
OR BLENDER AND SERVE. THIS MAKES TWO
LARGE GLASSES.

ACIA SUPER CHARGER

1 SMALL PACKAGE OF FROZEN ACIA BERRY
(YOU CAN PURCHASE THIS IN MOST SUPER
MARKETS OR HEALTH FOOD STORES)

2 CUPS SPINACH

1 CUP BLUEBERRIES

$\frac{1}{2}$ CUP ALMOND MILK

1 SMALL ORANGE
PEELED AND CUT INTO
QUARTERS

1 SCOOP OF RAW MEAL
REPLACEMENT

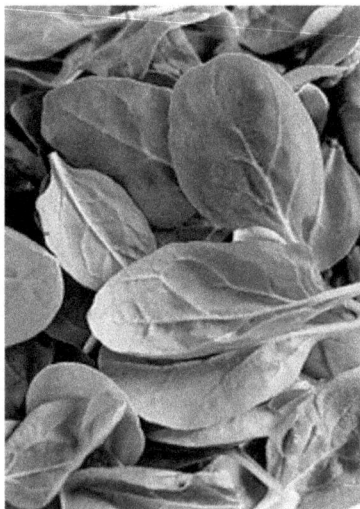

1 CUP OF ICE

1 TABLESPOON OF COCONUT OIL

1 PITTED DATE

MIX ALL INGREDIENTS IN A VITA MIXER
OR BLENDER AND SERVE. THIS MAKES 2
MEDIUM GLASSES.

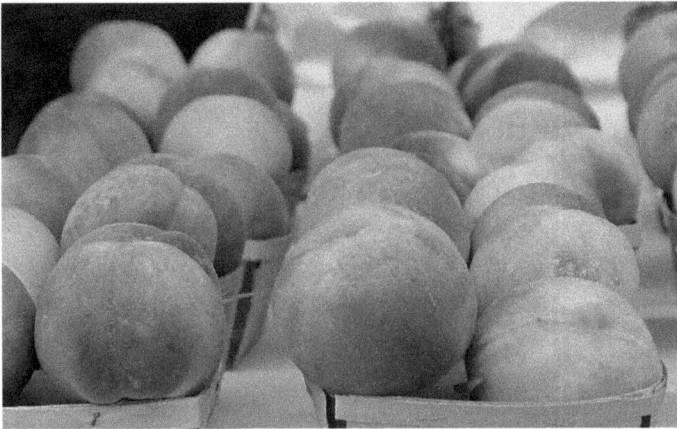

PEACHES & GREEN

2 SMALL PEACHES WITH THE PIT REMOVED
AND CUT INTO QUARTERS

2 CUP ROMAINE LETTUCE

1 CUP CELERY

¾ CUP OF ORANGE JUICE

1 SCOOP RAW MEAL REPLACEMENT

1 CUP OF ICE

MIX ALL INGREDIENTS IN A VITA MIXER OR A BLENDER AND SERVE. THIS MAKES TWO MEDIUM GLASSES.

GREEN APPLE

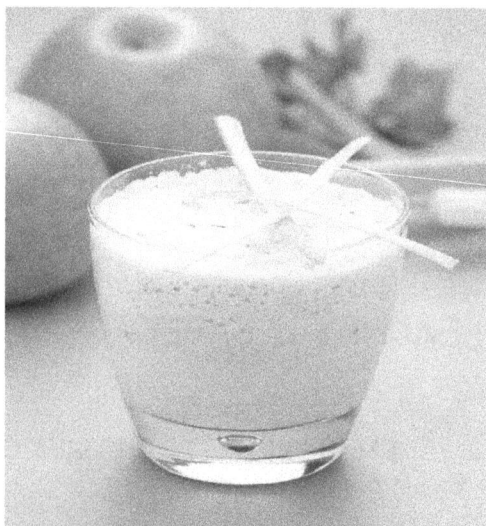

2 CUPS SPINACH

1 GREEN APPLE SEEDED AND CUT INTO QUARTERS

$\frac{1}{4}$ CUP LIME JUICE

1 CUP ALMOND MILK

1 SCOOP RAW MEAL REPLACEMENT

1 CUP OF ICE

MIX ALL INGREDIENTS IN A VITA MIXER OR BLENDER AND SERVE. THIS MAKES TWO SMALL GLASSES.

GREEN KIWI

1 CUP SPINACH

1 CUP CELERY

4 KIWIS PEELED AND CUT

$\frac{1}{2}$ CUP LIME JUICE

$\frac{1}{2}$ CUP ALMOND MILK

$\frac{1}{2}$ CUP ORANGE JUICE

1/8 CUP ALOE VERA JUICE

1 SCOOP RAW MEAL REPLACEMENT

1 CUP OF ICE

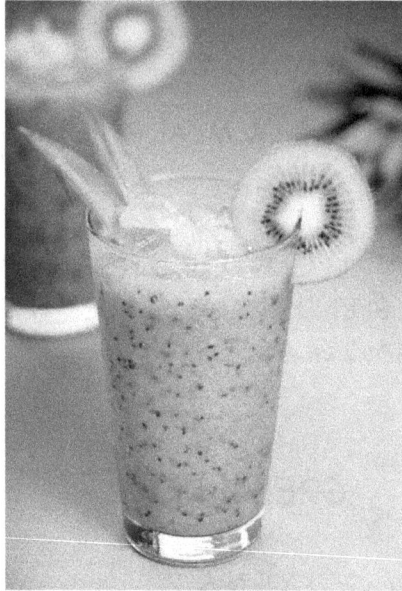

MIX ALL INGREDIENTS IN A VITA MIXER
OR BLENDER AND SERVE. THIS MAKES 2
MEDIUM GLASSES.

CUCUMBER MADNESS

1 LARGE CUCUMBER PEELED

1 HASS AVOCADO

$\frac{1}{4}$ CUP LIME JUICE

1 CUP WATER

1 CUP ICE

$\frac{1}{2}$ BUNCH OF FLAT LEAF PARSLEY

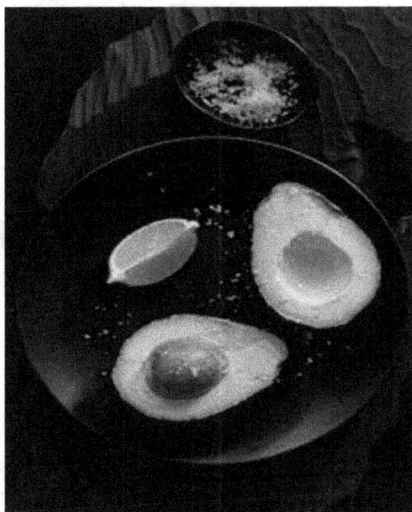

MIX ALL INGREDIENTS TOGETHER IN A VITA MIXER OR BLENDER AND SERVE. THIS MAKES TWO SMALL GLASSES.

CHOCOLATE HEAVEN

1 HASS AVOCADO (PITTED AND SLICED)

3 TABLESPOONS OF RAW COCOA POWDER

1 TABLESPOON OF AGAVE NECTAR

1 TABLESPOON OF COCONUT

2 DATES PITTED

2 CUPS ALMOND MILK

1 CUP OF ICE

1 FROZEN
BANANA

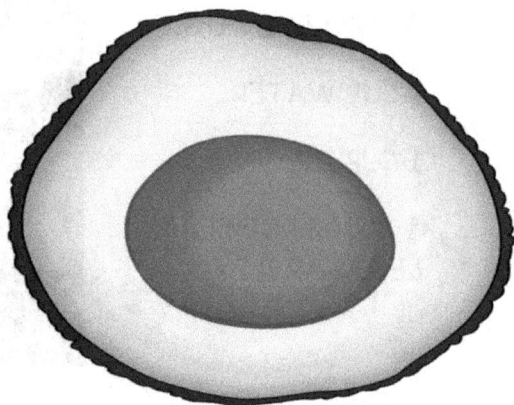

MIX ALL INGREDIENTS IN A VITAMIXER OR
BLENDER AND SERVE. THIS IS A GREAT
TREAT!

TROPICAL PAPAYA

1 $\frac{1}{2}$ CUPS PAPAYA

½ CUP PINEAPPLE

1 FROZEN BANANA

1 CUP COCONUT MILK

1 CUP ICE

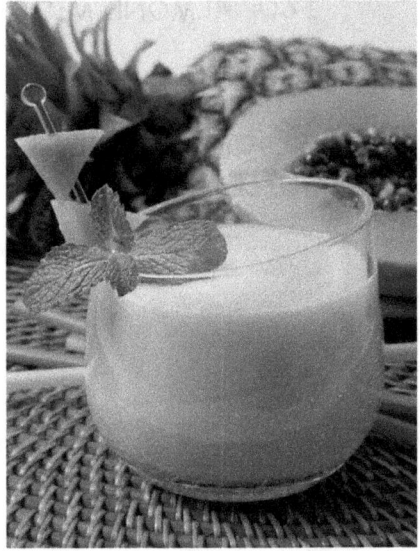

MIX ALL INGREDIENTS IN A VITA MIXER
OR BLENDER AND SERVE. THIS IS ANOTHER
YUMMY TREAT!

SWEET CHERRY

1 CUP FROZEN CHERRIES

2 CUPS ROMAINE LETTUCE

1 ORANGE PEELED AND CUT INTO QUARTERS

1 CUP ALMOND MILK

1 CUP ICE

SPLASH OF LIME
JUICE

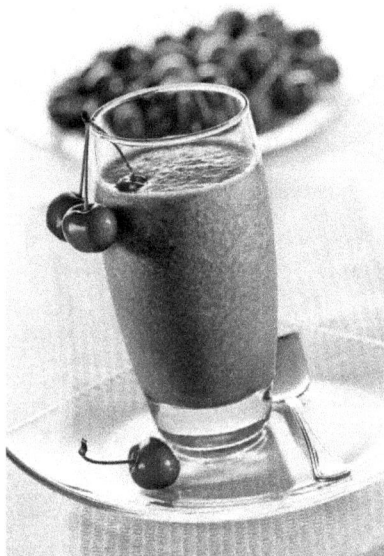

MIX ALL INGREDIENTS IN A VITA MIXER
OR BLENDER AND SERVE. THIS MAKES TWO
SMALL GLASSES.

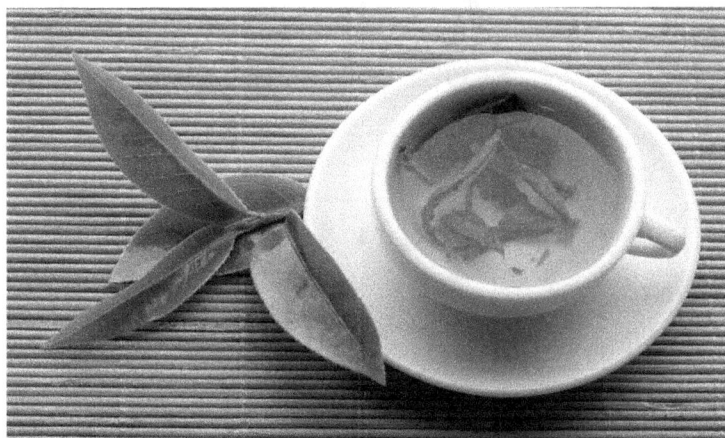

GREEN TEA SMOOTHIE

1 ½ CUPS OF CHILLED GREEN TEA

1 CUP ALMOND MILK

1 CUP OF ROMAINE LETTUCE

1 DATE PITTED

1 CUP OF ICE

MIX ALL INGREDIENTS IN A VITA MIXER
OR BLENDER AND SERVE. THIS IS A NICE
AND REFRESHING DRINK IN THE SUMMER!

BLUEBERRY GINGER SMOOTHIE

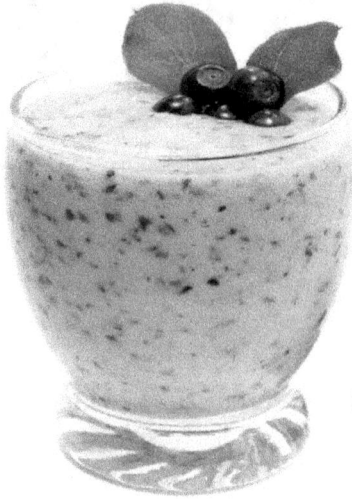

1 CUP OF BLUEBERRIES

½ APPLE (SEEDED AND SLICED)

2 ORANGES PEELED AND SLICED

1 GINGER TOE PEELED

½ CUP ALMOND MILK

1 CUP ROMAINE LETTUCE OR 3-4 STALKS

1 CUP OF ICE

MIX ALL INGREDIENTS IN A VITA MIXER OR A BLENDER AND SERVE. THIS MAKES 2 SMALL GLASSES. IF THIS IS TOO THICK YOU CAN ADD MORE ALMOND MILK OR WATER.

PEAR SMOOTHIE

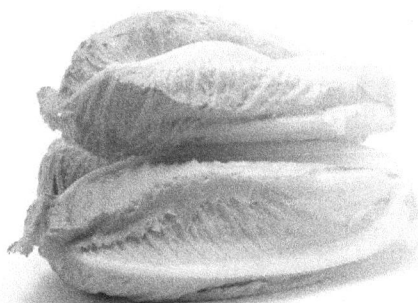

1 PEAR SLICED AND SEEDED

1 ORANGE PEELED AND CUT INTO QUARTERS

1 GINGER TOE PEELED

½ FROZEN BANANA

3-4 STALKS OF ROMAINE LETTUCE

1/2 CUP CELERY

1 CUP OF ALMOND MILK

1 CUP OF ICE

MIX ALL INGREDIENTS IN A VITA MIXER
OR BLENDER AND SERVE. THIS MAKES 2
SMALL GLASSES.

GREEN NECTARINE

5-6 ROMAINE STALKS

1/8 CUP OF ALOE VERA JUICE

1 CUP SPINACH

3 NECTARINES WITH THE SEED TAKEN OUT

2 DATES PITTED

SPLASH OF LIME JUICE

1 CUP OF ICE

1 CUP OF ALMOND MILK

MIX ALL INGREDIENTS IN A VITA MIXER
OR BLENDER AND SERVE. THIS MAKES 2
SMALL GLASSES.

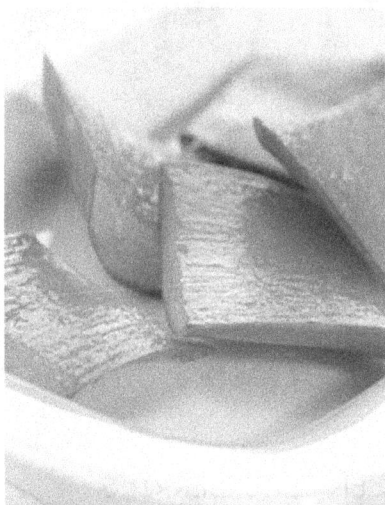

BLACKBERRY DREAM

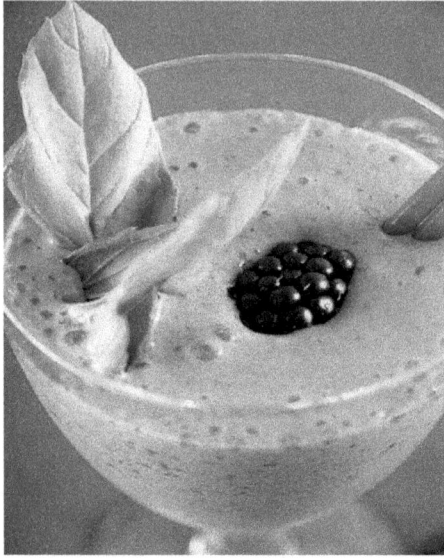

1 RAW COCONUT (SCOOP OUT THE INSIDE OF IT)

1 CUP FROZEN BLACKBERRIES

2 DATES PITTED

4-5 ROMAINE STALKS

½ FROZEN BANANA

1 CUP ALMOND MILK

1 CUP OF ICE

MIX ALL INGREDIENTS IN A VITA MIXER
OR BLENDER AND SERVE. THIS MAKES 2
MEDIUM GLASSES.

MIXED GREEN BERRY

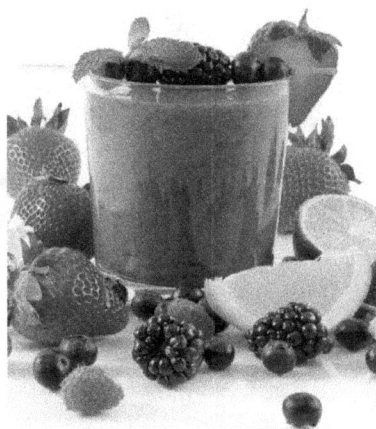

2 CUPS FROZEN MIXED BERRIES

3 CUPS OF SPINACH

$\frac{1}{2}$ FROZEN BANANA

1 CUP ALMOND MILK

1 CUP OF ICE

1/8 CUP OF LIME JUICE

1 TOE OF GINGER PEELED

MIX ALL INGREDIENTS IN A VITA MIXER
OR BLENDER AND SERVE. THIS MAKES TWO
MEDIUM GLASSES.

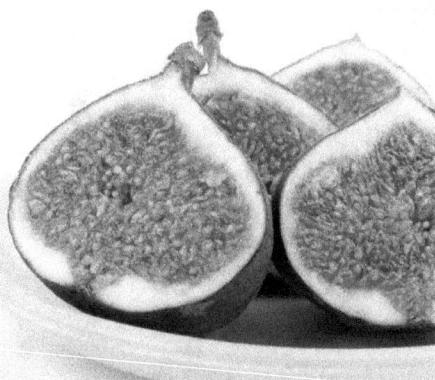

FIGLISIOUS

½ CUP BLUEBERRIES

3-4 FIGS

1 DATE PITTED

2 CUPS OF SPINACH

1 ORANGE PEELED AND QUARTERED

1 CUP ALMOND MILK

1 CUP OF ICE

MIX ALL INGREDIENTS IN A VITA MIXER
OR BLENDER AND SERVE. THIS MAKES 2
SMALL GLASSES.

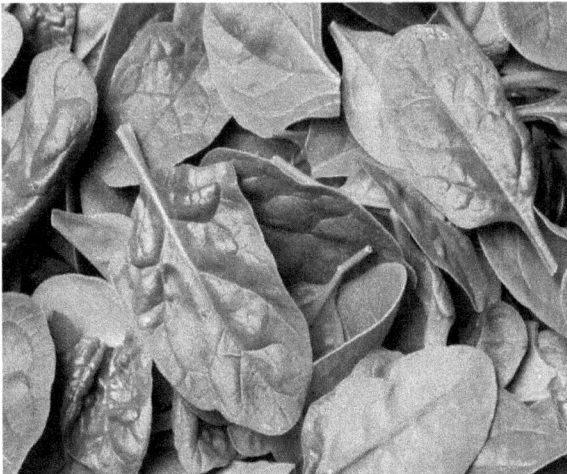

20 Raw Soups

CREAMY AVOCADO AND CUCUMBER MEDLEY

MACHO GAZPACHO

CREAMY RED PEPPER SOUP

CREAMY PEA SOUP

CREAMY CARROT FENNEL SOUP

THAI COCONUT LEMON GRASS SOUP

SPICY WATERMELON TOMATO SOUP

CREAMY CELERY AND GREEN APPLE SOUP

RAW CREAMY CELERY SOUP

RAW TOMATO SOUP

SUN DRIED TOMATO AND POBLANO CHILI SOUP

CREAMY BUTTERNUT SQUASH SOUP

SPINACH SOUP

SWEET SUMMER WATERMELON SOUP

MANGO/MADNESS

PEANUT SOUP

BLACK PEPPER AND ZUCCHINI SOUP

COCONUT AND MACADAMIA NUT SOUP

SUMMER ROMAINE SOUP

KALE NUTRITION SOUP

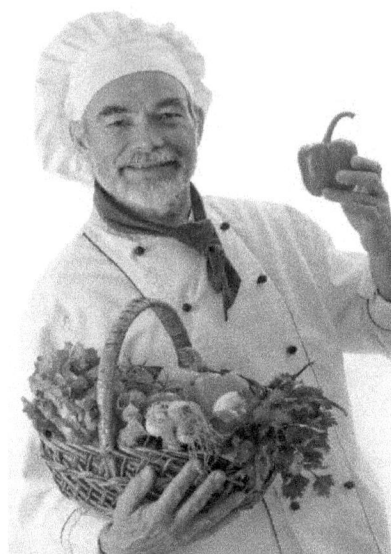

CREAMY AVOCADO AND CUCUMBER MEDLEY

4 LARGE ORGANIC CUCUMBERS, PEELED
4 ORGANIC CELERY STALKS

2 HASS AVOCADOS PEELED AND PITTED
2 LIMES
4 CUPS PURIFIED WATER

PUT ALL THE INGREDIENTS IN THE VITA-
MIXER AND CHILL AND SERVE GARNISHED WITH
CILANTRO SPRIGS! YUM!

MACHO GAZPACHO

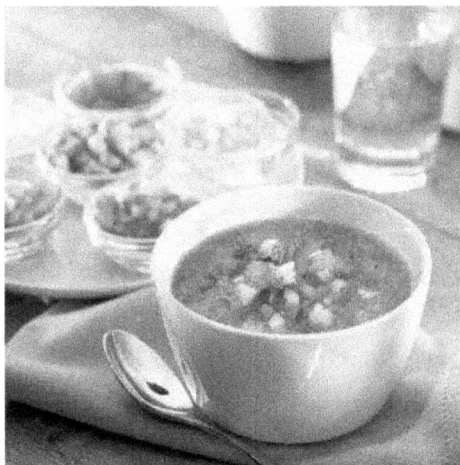

4 CUPS ROMA TOMATOES
1 CUP DICED AND SEEDED TOMATOES
1 CUP PEELED, SEEDED CUCUMBER DICED

2 Cup Red, Green, and Yellow
Peppers
2 Limes squeezed into soup
2 Avocados cut into small pieces
3 Cloves of garlic crushed
1 Small bunch of Cilantro chopped
1 Small jalapeno, seeded and
minced
1/2 Green onion minced
1 Teaspoon sea salt
Fresh Ground Black pepper

Puree the 4 cups of roma tomatoes
and then add all the other
ingredients and voila' you have
Macho Gazpacho!

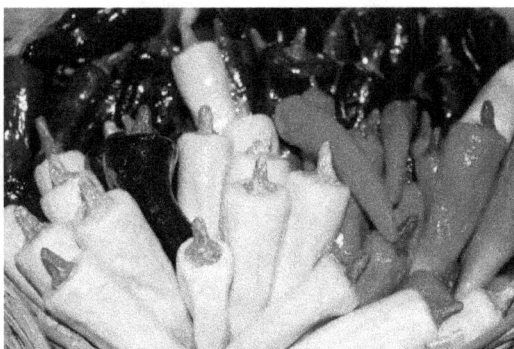

CREAMY RED PEPPER SOUP

3 ORGANIC RED BELL PEPPERS SEEDED AND
STEMS REMOVED
1 YOUNG COCONUT
2 CLOVES OF GARLIC
3 TABLESPOONS COLD PRESSED EXTRA VIRGIN
OLIVE OIL
1 BUNCH OF ORGANIC CILANTRO
2 TEASPOONS OF SEA SALT
2 LIMES SQUEEZED

IF YOU LIKE IT SPICIER YOU CAN ADD A
JALAPENO OR SOME CAYENNE PEPPER IT JUST
DEPENDS ON HOW HOT YOU LIKE IT.

USE ALL THE COCONUT MEAT AND JUICE. THEN MIX ALL THE INGREDIENTS IN A VITA-MIXER EXCEPT HALF OF THE CILANTRO (USE THE REST AS A GARNISH) AND YOU HAVE RED PEPPER SOUP. THIS IS A GREAT SOUP FOR BOOSTING YOUR VITAMIN C INTAKE SO EAT UP!

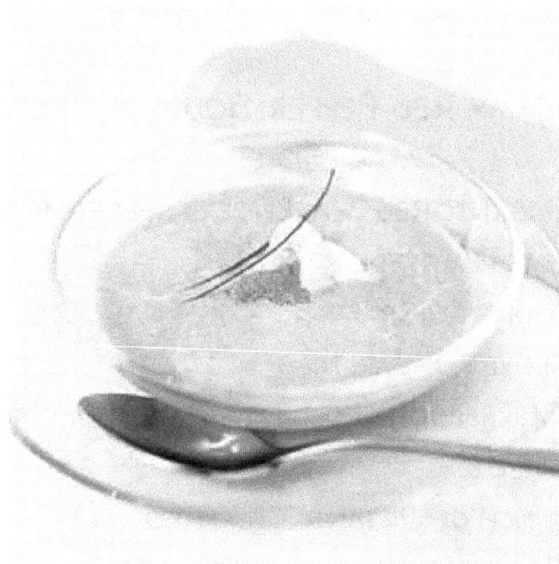

CREAMY PEA SOUP

2 CUPS ORGANIC FRESH PEAS
2 CUPS OF PURIFIED WATER

1 LARGE RIPE AVOCADO

1 BUNCH BASIL LEAVES

3 CLOVES OF ORGANIC GARLIC

1 TEASPOON OF SEA SALT

BLEND ALL INGREDIENTS IN A VITA MIXER AND BLEND UNTIL SMOOTH!

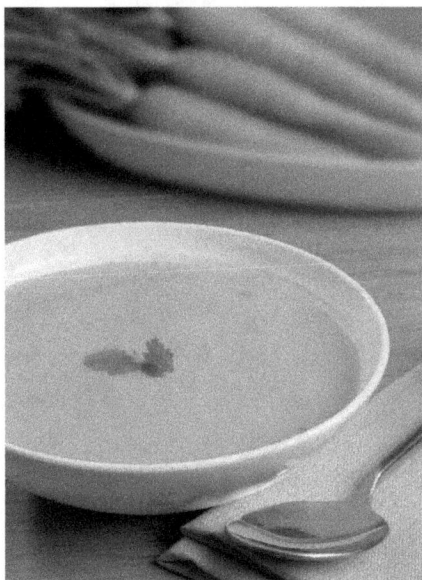

CREAMY CARROT FENNEL SOUP

4 CUPS OF PURIFIED WATER

4 ORGANIC CARROTS

1 LARGE AVOCADO

1 ORGANIC APPLE OF YOUR CHOICE

1 LARGE FENNEL BULB CHOPPED

1 TEASPOON OF SEA SALT

2 TABLESPOONS OF DILL WEED

BLEND ALL INGREDIENTS IN A VITA-MIXER UNTIL CREAMY AND ENJOY!

THAI COCONUT LEMON GRASS SOUP

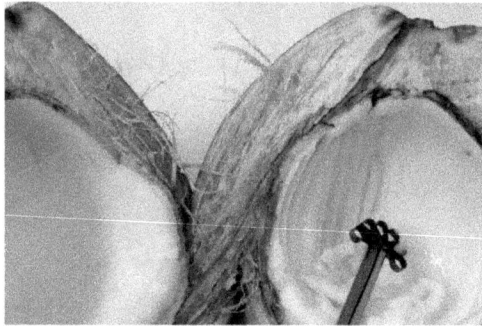

2 CUPS YOUNG COCONUT MEAT

2 CUPS COCONUT WATER

3 TABLESPOONS OF GINGER

1 TABLESPOON THAI CHILI PASTE

2 CLOVES OF GARLIC

1 Bunch of Organic Cilantro

2 Tablespoon of ground lemon grass

1/2 Bunch of Italian Parsley

3 Tablespoons of Cold Pressed Olive Oil

3 Tablespoons Tamari

Sea Salt to your tasting

Blend all ingredients in the Vita-mixer
and there you have a great healthy meal!

Spicy Watermelon Tomato Soup

4 Cups Watermelon seeded

2 cups any kind of Tomatoes

1 Cup Diced Tomatoes

1 Cup Diced Peeled Cucumber

1 Cup Diced Green and Red Peppers

1/4-1/2 (Depending on your tastes I like
a lot of lime) Cup Key Lime Juice

1 Large Jalapeño Diced Into Small Pieces

1 Large Bunch of Cilantro chopped fine

1 Large Piece of Ginger peeled

Salt and Pepper to taste

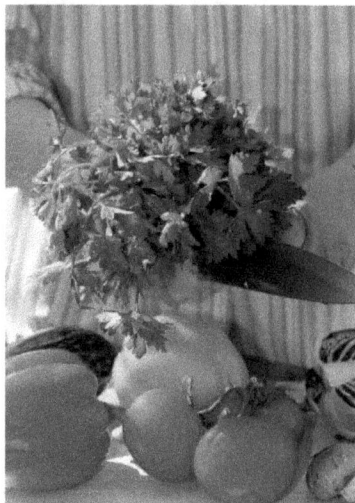

First puree the 4 cups of watermelon and 2 cups of tomatoes along with the ginger in a Vita-Mixer. Then add all the other diced ingredients and eat up! This is great for summer or really anytime. It is very refreshing chilled!

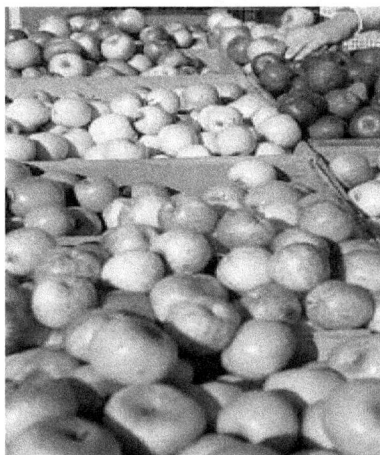

Creamy Celery and Green Apple Soup

1 Bunch Organic Celery
4 Large Organic Granny Smith Apples
1/4 -1/2 Cup Lemon Juice (depends on your taste)
1/4 Cup Cold Pressed Olive Oil
2 Tablespoons of Coconut Butter (this you can find at most health food stores)
2 Cups Soaked Raw Macadamia nuts (soak for at least 2 hours)
1 Cup Water or to your thickness
See Salt and Black Pepper to taste
You can add chopped parsley for a garnish or even both red and green apples mixed

71

TO GIVE IT A NICE COLOR.

THIS IS A BIT OF A LABOR OF LOVE SOUP BUT IT IS VERY TASTY! FIRST CUT THE CELERY INTO SMALL PIECES AND ONLY 3 OF THE GRANNY SMITH APPLES AND PUT INTO THE VITA MIXER.

ONCE THIS IS DONE DRAIN THE JUICE FROM THE PULP AND SAVE BOTH. NOW WASH THE SOAKED MACADAMIA NUTS AND THROW THEM IN THE VITA MIXER ALONG WITH THE STRAINED JUICE, WATER, OLIVE OIL, LEMON JUICE, AND S & P IF YOU WANT A THICKER SOUP YOU CAN ADD BACK SOME OF THE PULP. NOW THAT THIS IS DONE YOU GARNISH WITH THE LAST GRANNY SMITH APPLE THAT YOU CUT INTO SMALL BITES SIZE PIECES AND SERVE. YOU CAN ADD WHITE TRUFFLE OIL FOR AN EVEN RICHER SOUP OR IF YOU ARE HAVING QUESTS DUE TO THE PRICE OF THE OIL.

RAW CREAMY CELERY SOUP

1 BUNCH OF CELERY
1/2 CUP OLIVE OIL
1/4 CUP LEMON JUICE

4 CUPS OF WATER

2 TEASPOONS OF AGAVE NECTAR

1 CUP SOAKED RAW CASHEWS

3/4 CUP OF PARSLEY

YOU CAN ALSO TOP THIS SOUP OFF WITH CHOPPED AVOCADO, SLICED CARROTS, OR CHOPPED RED PEPPER AND PARSLEY.

BLEND ALL INGREDIENTS IN A VITA MIXER UNTIL SMOOTH AND CREAMY. IF YOU WANT THE SOUP THICKER JUST USE 1 CUP LESS WATER IN THE RECIPE. THIS IS GREAT SOUP FOR THE SUMMER CHILLED OR RIGHT OUT OF THE VITA MIXER!

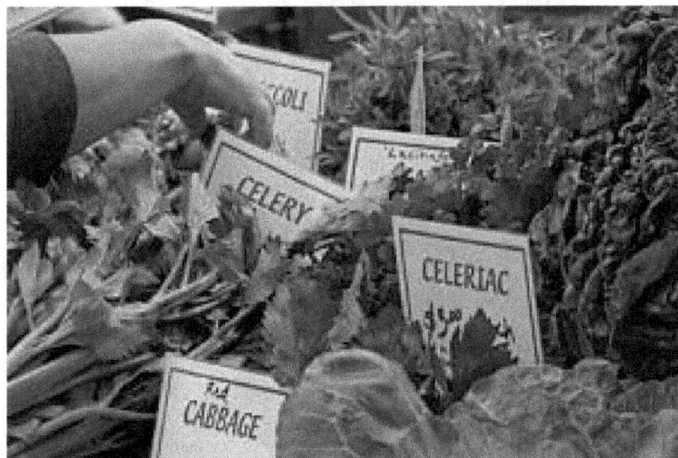

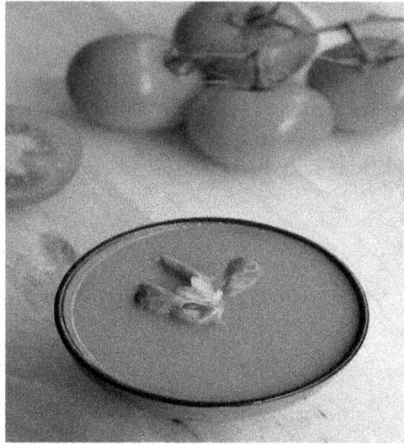

Raw Tomato Soup

8 Large Tomatoes
2 Cloves of Garlic peeled
¼ Cup of Lime Juice
1/8 Cup of Olive Oil
Salt and Pepper to your liking
Tablespoon of Chopped Basil
Tablespoon of Chopped Oregano

This is one of the easiest raw soups to make! Just blend all ingredients with a Vita mixer until smooth consistency and garnish with a few basil sprigs!

Sun Dried Tomato and Poblano Chili Soup (this is a hot one)

1 Cup of sun dried tomatoes Soaked for 4-5 hours

2-3 Dried Poblanos soaked for 4-5 hours

3 Cups of Water

$\frac{1}{2}$ Cup of Lemon Juice

$\frac{1}{4}$ Cup of Olive Oil

1 small peeled cucumber

Chopped Parsley

Chopped Cilantro

Salt and Pepper to taste

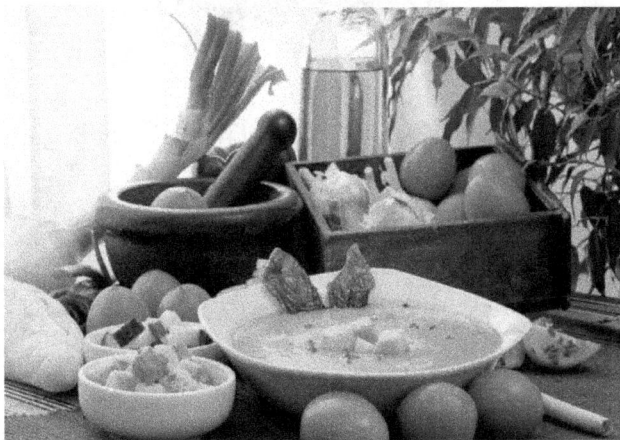

RINSE THE SOAKED TOMATOES AND POBLANO CHILIES AND PUT THEM ALONG WITH THE REST OF THE INGREDIENTS IN THE VITA MIXER AND GARNISH WITH CILANTRO AND EXTRA SLICE OF LEMONS OR LIMES!

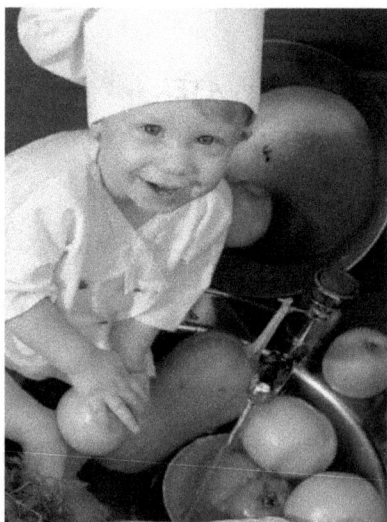

CREAMY BUTTERNUT SQUASH SOUP

3 CUPS PEELED AND CUT INTO SMALLER PIECES FOR THE VITA MIXER

1/8 CUP OLIVE OIL

1/8 CUP OF RAW PEANUT BUTTER

2 TABLESPOONS OF PARSLEY

1 TEASPOON OF CURRY POWDER

¼ LIME JUICE

¾ CUP OF WATER

SEA SALT OF BRAGGS TO YOUR LIKING

1 TABLESPOON OF AGAVE NECTAR

MIX ALL OF THE ABOVE INGREDIENTS INTO A VITA MIXER UNTIL SMOOTH AND GARNISH WITH FRESH PARSLEY SPRIGS!

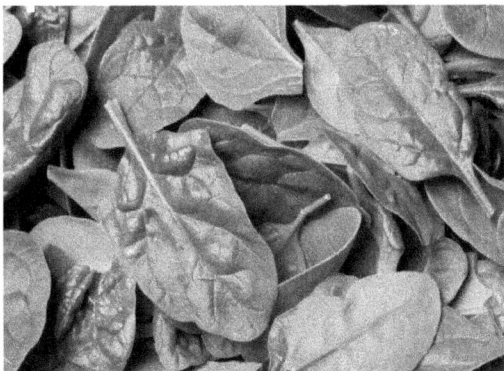

SPINACH SOUP

1 CUP OF ALMOND MILK

1 CUP OF WATER

5 CUPS OF SPINACH

2 SMALL CUCUMBERS PEELED

1 CLOVE OF GARLIC

$\frac{1}{4}$ CUP OF ALMOND BUTTER

1/8 CUP OF LIME JUICE

1/8 CUP OF HEMP OIL

SALT AND PEPPER TO TASTE OR BRAGGS IF YOU LIKE

MIX ALL INGREDIENTS IN THE VITA MIXER AND GARNISH WITH A FEW SLICES OF CUCUMBER!

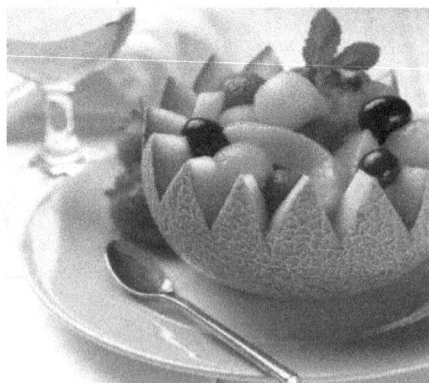

SWEET SUMMER WATERMELON SOUP

6 CUPS OF WATERMELON

1 CUP HONEY DEW MELLON

1 CUP OF ICE
½ CUP OF PINEAPPLE JUICE
CHOPPED MINT

MIX ALL INGREDIENTS IN A VITA MIXER EXCEPT 1 CUP OF THE WATERMELON (CUT INTO SMALL CHUNKS AND USE AS A GARNISH)! THIS IS A GREAT SOUP TO COOL YOU OFF IN THE SUMMER!

MANGO MADNESS

4 LARGE RIPE MANGOES PEELED AND CUT INTO PIECES (JUST SO THAT THE MANGO FLESH IS SEPARATED FROM THE SEED)
¼ CUP LIME JUICE
2 CUP ORANGE JUICE
3 PITTED DATES
CHOPPED MINT

MIX ALL INGREDIENTS EXCEPT ONE OF THE MANGOES (SAVE IT FOR GARNISH IN THE SOUP) IN A VITA MIXER AND GARNISH WITH THE EXTRA MANGO AND CHOPPED MINT!

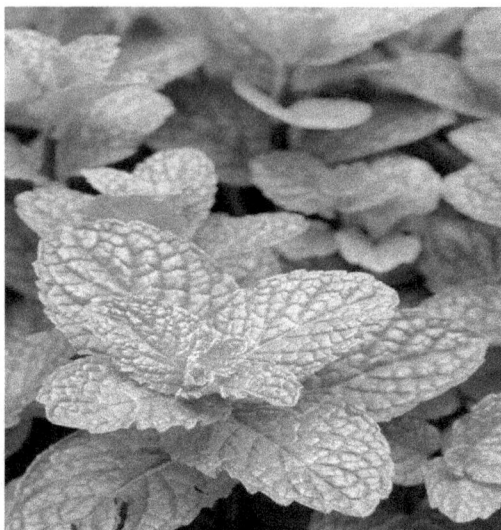

Peanut Soup

2 Cups Water

1 Cup Orange Juice

2 Ripe Bananas

1 Teaspoon Curry Powder

1 Cup natural Peanut butter

$\frac{1}{4}$ cup Lime juice

1 Tablespoon peeled ginger root

1 Clove of garlic

Chopped Cilantro

MIX ALL INGREDIENTS EXCEPT THE CILANTRO IN A VITA MIXER AND BLEND UNTIL SMOOTH. GARNISH WITH CHOPPED PEANUTS AND CHOPPED CILANTRO! YUM!

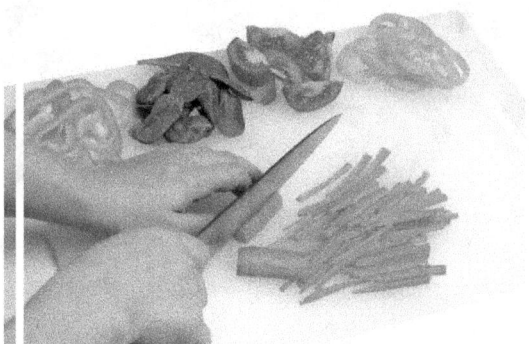

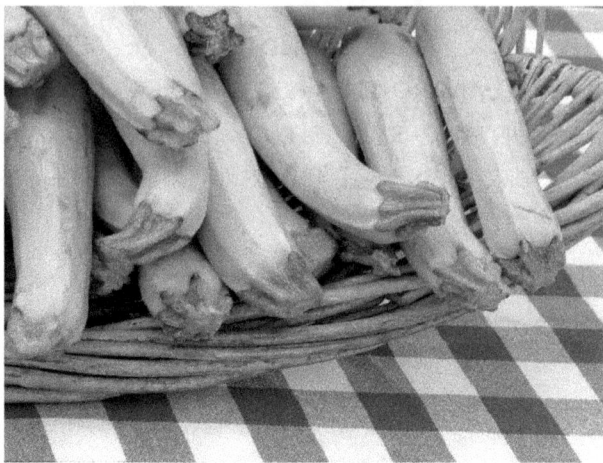

BLACK PEPPER AND ZUCCHINI SOUP

4 PEELED ZUCCHINIS

4 STALKS OF CELERY

2 CUPS OF WATER

$\frac{1}{4}$ CUP OF OLIVE OIL

1 TABLESPOON OF BLACK PEPPER

1 CLOVE OF GARLIC

SALT TO TASTE

BLEND ALL INGREDIENTS IN A VITA MIXER AND GARNISH WITH MORE BLACK PEPPER! SPICY BUT GOOD!

Coconut and Macadamia Nut soup

2 Cups raw macadamia nuts soaked
for several hours
1 raw coconut Scooped and the
water saved
2 cups extra coconut water
$\frac{1}{4}$ lime juice
1/8 cup of macadamia nut oil
Salt and Pepper to taste
Cilantro for garnish

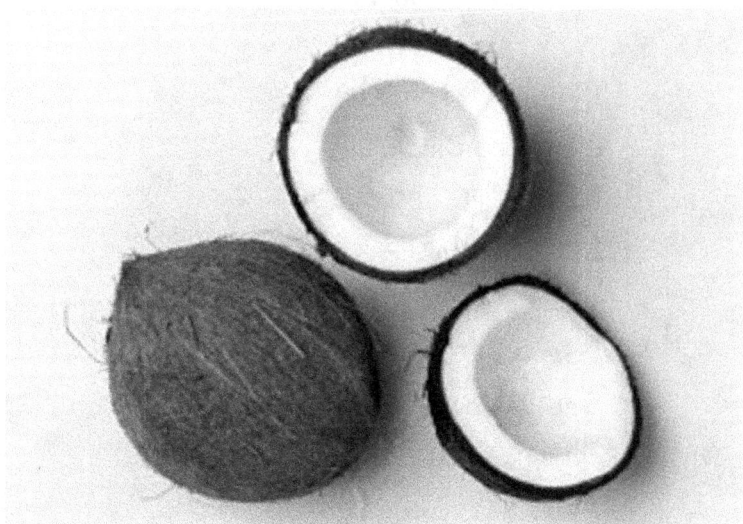

Drain the soaked macadamia nuts and put the rest of the ingredients in the Vita mixer and blend until smooth. Garnish with chopped macadamia nuts, raw shredded coconut, and cilantro! Yum you will have more friends than you want with this soup!

Summer Romaine Soup

1 head of romaine lettuce

2 stalks of celery

1 small peeled cucumber

1 cup of water

$\frac{1}{4}$ cup lemon juice

1 small piece of ginger peeled

Salt and pepper to taste

Garnish with chopped cilantro

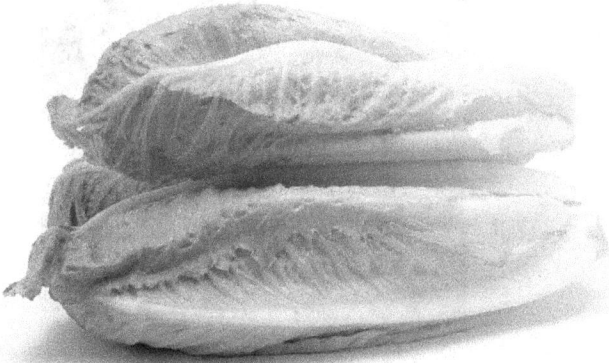

BLEND ALL INGREDIENTS IN A VITA
MIXER AND BLEND UNTIL SMOOTH.
GARNISH WITH CHOPPED CILANTRO!
THIS IS A NICE A REFRESHING SUMMER
SOUP!

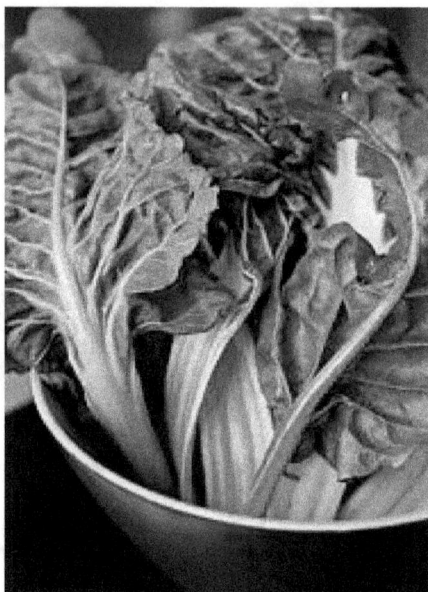

KALE NUTRITION SOUP

6 CUPS OF KALE

2 CUPS OF WATER

1 PEELED CUCUMBER

$\frac{1}{4}$ CUP OF LEMON JUICE

1/8 CUP OF OLIVE OIL

$\frac{1}{2}$ CUP OF FLAT LEAF PARSLEY

3 CELERY STALKS

SALT AND PEPPER TO TASTE

MIX ALL INGREDIENTS TOGETHER IN A VITA MIXER AND BLEND UNTIL SMOOTH. THE CONSISTENCY WILL BE A LITTLE ON THE THICKER SIDE AND GARNISH WITH CHOPPED CUCUMBERS! THIS IS DELISH AND NUTRISH!

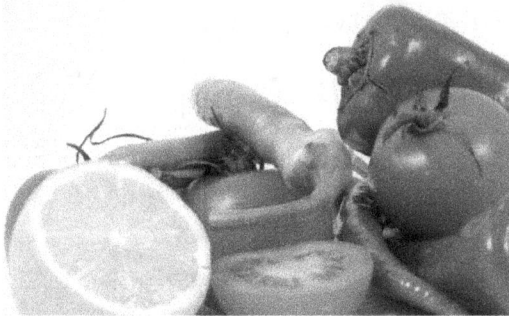

20 Raw Main Dishes

COLLARD WRAPS

CRUNCHY LETTUCE WRAPS

SWEET NORI WRAPS

VEGGIE NORI WRAPS

SUN DRIED TOMATO & ARUGULA PIZZA

MUSHROOM & TOMATO PESTO PIZZA

MEDITERRANEAN BURRITOS

ALFREDO RAW PASTA

PESTO LINGUINI

SPAGHETTI SQUASH PASTA & SPICY

GARLIC SAUCE

ITALIAN CAPRESE TOWERS

LASAGNA

STUFFED TOMATOES

RAWVIOLI

QUINOA SUMMER SALAD

THAI WILD RICE SALAD

SWEET SUMMER WILD RICE SALAD

RAW BURGER

LENTIL SALAD

ITALIAN BARLEY SALAD

COLLARD WRAPS

6 MEDIUM COLLARD LEAVES (WASHED
WITH THE STEM TAKEN OFF IF THEY ARE
TOO LONG)
1CUP SHREDDED CARROTS
1 CUP 1 INCH THINLY SLICED CUCUMBERS
1 CUP THINLY SLICED RED PEPPERS
1 CUP SPROUTS
$\frac{1}{4}$ CUP RAW SUNFLOWER SEEDS
$\frac{1}{2}$ CUP OF SOME TYPE OF SPREAD LIKE RAW
PESTO, RAW SUNDRIED TOMATO SPREAD,
HUMMUS (WHATEVER ONE YOU LIKE THE
BEST)

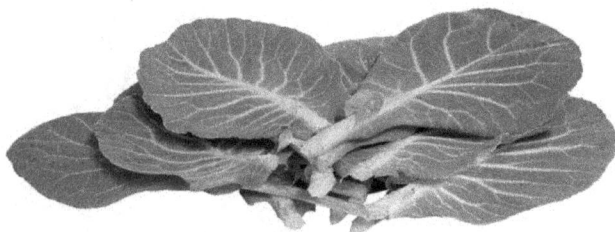

TAKE THE WASHED COLLARD GREENS AND
LAY THEM FLAT. FIRST PUT THE SPREAD OF
YOUR CHOICE IN THE MIDDLE OF THE LEAF
THEN PUT SOME OF EACH OF THE REST OF
THE INGREDIENTS AND WRAP LIKE A
BURRITO! YUM THESE ARE SO GOOD AND
GOOD FOR YOU TOO!

CRUNCHY LETTUCE WRAPS

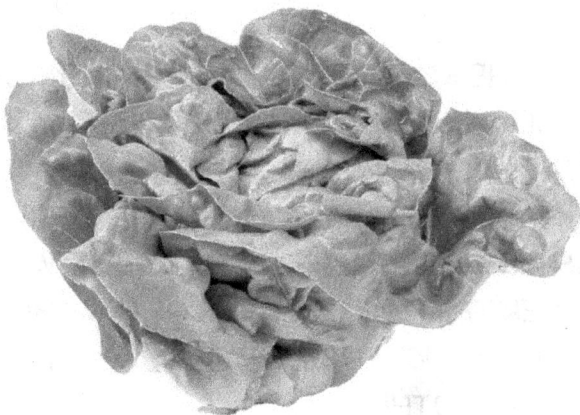

A SMALL HEAD OF BIB LETTUCE OR
ROMAINE (CLEANED AND WASHED)
1 CUP JICAMA (PEELED AND SLICED INTO
THIN 1 INCH PIECES)
½ CUP CILANTRO CLEANED (NOT CHOPPED;
JUST KEPT IN SINGLE STRANDS)
1 CUP THINLY SLICED RED PEPPERS
2 CUP OF BEAN SPROUTS
1/2 CUP CHOPPED RAW PEANUTS (FOR TOP)
½ CUP LIME PEANUT SAUCE (THIS IS A
SIMPLE SAUCE OF RAW PEANUT BUTTER
MIXED WITH LIME JUICE TO THE
CONSISTENCY OF A THIN SAUCE)

TAKE THE BIB LETTUCE OR ROMAINE (I LIKE
BIB BECAUSE IT IS A LITTLE SOFTER AND
EASIER TO HANDLE WHEN YOU ARE EATING
IT) AND PUT SOME OF EACH INGREDIENT
INSIDE AND WRAP IT UP AND SERVE WITH
EITHER THE PEANUT SAUCE OR PUT THE
PEANUT SAUCE INSIDE THE WRAP. I LIKE
IT WITH BOTH!

SWEET NORI WRAPS

1 CUP STRAWBERRIES THINLY SLICED
1 CUP PAPAYA THINLY SLICED
1 CUP MANGO THINLY SLICED
¼ CUP MINT LEAVES WHOLE
CASHEW DIPPING SAUCE, WHICH IS 1 CUP
CASHEWS SOAKED FOR 4 HOURS AND THEN
DRAINED. PUT THE SOAKED CASHEWS
INTO A VITAMIXER ALONG WITH 2
TABLESPOONS OF LIME JUICE, AND 1
TABLESPOON OF AGAVE NECTAR, AND A
SMALL AMOUNT OF WATER OR ½ AN
ORANGE SQUEEZED TO MAKE THE RIGHT
CONSISTENCY FOR A SAUCE.

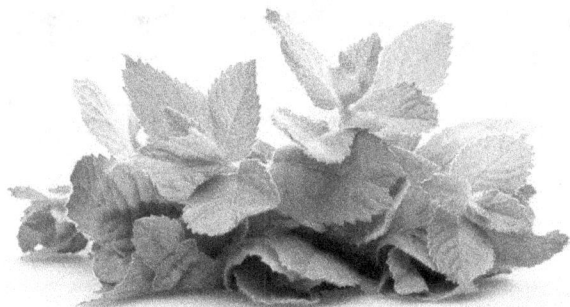

KEEP THE NORI SHEETS DRY ON A CUTTING
BOARD AND START TO FILL THE NORI AT
THE END THAT IS CLOSEST TO YOU WITH
THE FRUITS AND THEN START ROLLING
THE NORI UP. AFTER THAT YOU WILL SLICE
THE NORI INTO SMALLER SUSHI STYLE
PIECES AND DIP THE PIECES INTO THE
DIPPING SAUCE.

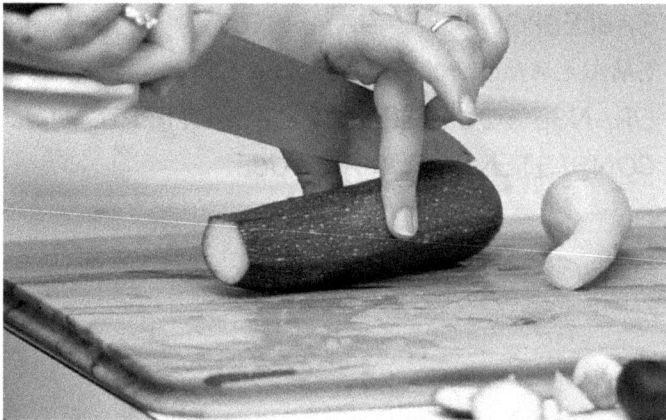

VEGGIE NORI WRAPS

1 CUP THINLY SLICED ZUCCHINI
1 CUP THINLY SLICED CARROTS
1 CUP THINLY SLICED RED PEPPER

2 AVOCADOS
1 CUP THINLY SLICED CUCUMBER
1 CUP OF BASIL LEAVES

TAKE THE VEGETABLES AND CLEAN AND
PEEL THEM THEN TAKE THE CARROT, RED
PEPPER, AND CUCUMBER AND MAKE THIN
SLICES THE LENGTH OF THE VEGETABLE.
TAKE THE AVOCADOS AND DESEED THEM
AND MASH THEM UP INTO A SPREAD.

AGAIN KEEP THE NORI SHEETS DRY AND
START AND THE END CLOSEST TO YOU AND
PUT A THIN LAYER OF THE AVOCADO
SPREAD ON THE BEGINNING OF THE NORI
SHEET, THEN SOME OF EACH OF THE OTHER
VEGGIES AND THEN ROLL IT, SLICE IT, AND
EAT IT! YOU CAN USE BRAGGS FOR A
DIPPING SAUCE IF YOU LIKE OR WHATEVER
YOU LIKE BEST.

SUN DRIED TOMATO & ARUGULA PIZZA

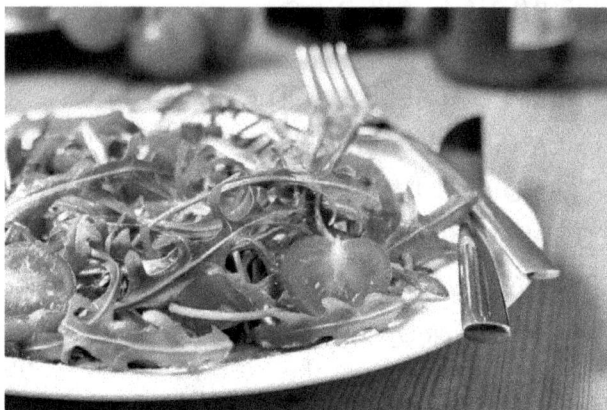

2 CUPS OF ARUGULA
1 CUP SUNDRIED TOMATO SPREAD (WHICH
IS ¾ CUP OF SUNDRIED TOMATOES SOAKED
AND DRAINED. USING A VITAMIXER GRIND
UP THE SUNDRIED TOMATOES ALONG WITH
¼ CUP OLIVE OIL, SALT AND PEPPER, ¼ CUP
RAW PINE NUTS & HALF OF THE BASIL)
4-5 SEED, FLAX, ETC DEHYDRATED CRACKERS
OF YOUR LIKING. YOU CAN PURCHASE
THESE IN MOST HEALTH FOOD STORES OR
IF YOU FEEL AMBITIOUS YOU CAN ALSO
MAKE THEM YOURSELF!
¼ CUP BASIL

TAKE THE FLAX CRACKERS AND SPREAD THE
SUNDRIED TOMATO SPREAD ON THE TOP.
TAKE THE ARUGULA AND THE REST OF THE
BASIL AND MIX IT WITH A LITTLE
BALSAMIC AND OLIVE OIL (JUST ENOUGH
TO BARELY COAT THE ARUGULA) AND THEN
PUT THE ARUGULA ON TOP OF THE SUN
DRIED TOMATO SPREAD AND YOUR DONE!
THIS IS A GREAT TREAT. YOU CAN ALSO
USE OTHER ITEMS LIKE TOMATOES SLICED,
GREEN PEPPERS, RED PEPPERS, ETC.

MUSHROOM & TOMATO PESTO PIZZA

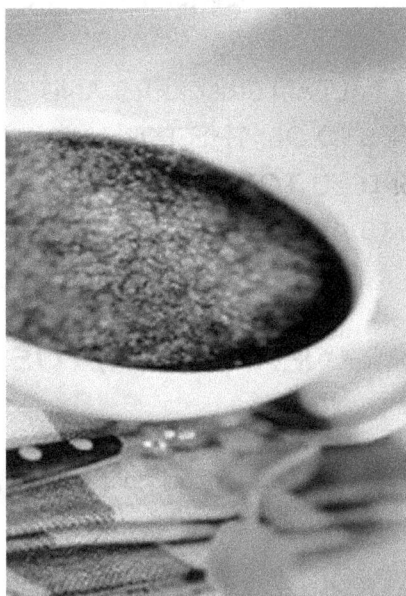

4-5 FLAX, ITALIAN, ETC DEHYDRATED
CRACKERS
PESTO SAUCE (1 CUP WALNUTS SOAKED FOR
4-5 HOURS AND DRAINED, 1 CUP BASIL
LEAVES, ¼-1/2 CUP OF OLIVE OIL, 1/8 CUP
LIME JUICE 1 CLOVE OF GARLIC AND SALT
AND PEPPER TO TASTE. USING THE
VITAMIXER GRIND ALL OF THE
INGREDIENTS TOGETHER TO A SMOOTH
CONSISTENCY (YOU MAY NEED A LITTLE
WATER OR EXTRA OLIVE OIL IT WILL JUST
DEPEND).
1 CUP SLICED TOMATOES
1 CUP SLICED CRIMINI MUSHROOMS

TAKE THE ITALIAN CRACKERS AND SPREAD
THE RAW PESTO ON THE TOP AND THEN
ADD THE SLICED TOMATOES AND
MUSHROOMS AND SPRINKLE WITH BASIL.

MEDITERRANEAN BURRITOS

2 CUPS SPROUTED GARBANZO BEANS (SEE
MY WEBSITE
WWW.RAWFOODFORTODAY.COM) OR SOAK

THE BEANS FOR 8 HOURS AND ALLOW TO
SPROUT FOR 2-3 DAYS
1/2 CUP OLIVE OIL
¼ CUP RAW TAHINI BUTTER

6-8 BIB LETTUCE LEAVES NOT BROKEN
1 CUP SLICED CUCUMBERS IN 1 INCH PIECES
1 CUP RED PEPPERS SLICED INTO 1 INCH
PIECES
1 CUP DICED TOMATOES
1 BUNCH OF CHOPPED CILANTRO
SALT AND PEPPER

IN A FOOD PROCESSOR COMBINE
GARBANZO BEANS, TAHINI BUTTER, OLIVE
OIL, AND SALT AND PEPPER AND BLEND
UNTIL SMOOTH. NEXT SPREAD THE
GARBANZO BEAN MIXTURE ON THE INSIDE
OF THE BIB LETTUCE AND ARRANGE THE
RAW VEGGIES AND WRAP IT UP AND EAT IT!
THIS IS GREAT BECAUSE YOU CAN PUT ALL
KINDS OF VEGGIES IN THESE AND CHANGE
IT UP A LITTLE MORE.

ALFREDO RAW PASTA

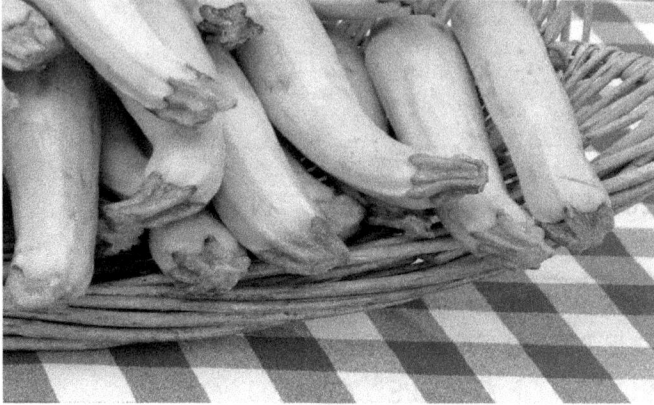

3-4 MEDIUM YELLOW ZUCCHINI USE A
SPIRAL SLICER AND SLICE ALL OF THE
ZUCCHINI INTO LONG SPIRALS

2 CUPS OF RAW CASHEWS SOAKED FOR 4-6
HOURS
$\frac{1}{4}$ CUP OLIVE OIL
1 CLOVE OF GARLIC
$\frac{1}{2}$ CUP OF LEMON JUICE
SALT AND PEPPER
$\frac{1}{4}$ CUP OF BASIL
1/8 CUP OF BRAGGS AMINO ACIDS

THIS IS ONE OF MY FAVORITE MEALS! I
LOVE THIS! ONCE YOU HAVE THE ZUCCHINI
SLICED PUT IT IN A LARGE BOWL. NOW
TAKE THE SOAKED CASHEWS AND DRAIN
THEM AND PUT THE CASHEWS AND THE
REST OF THE INGREDIENTS INTO A
VITAMIXER AND BLEND UNTIL IT IS A
SMOOTH SAUCE. NEXT PUT THE SAUCE ON
THE ZUCCHINI AND SPRINKLE WITH BASIL.

PESTO LINGUINI

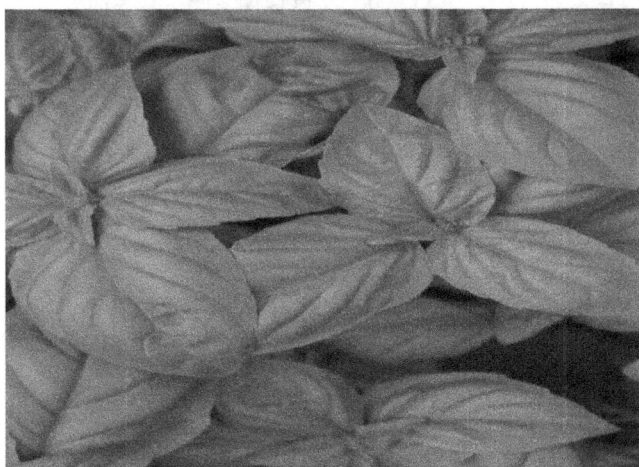

3-4 ZUCCHINI OR SQUASH

2 CUPS RAW WALNUTS NUTS SOAKED FOR
4-6 HOURS

1 ½ CUPS OF BASIL
½ CUP OIL
SALT AND PEPPER
CLOVE OF GARLIC

START WITH TAKING THE ZUCCHINI OR
SQUASH AND CUTTING IT INTO A LARGE
SQUARE BY CUTTING THE SKIN OFF. THEN
CUT THAT IN HALF AND TAKE A PEELER AND
MAKE STRIPS OUT OF BOTH HALVES SO
THAT THEY LOOK LIKE FETTUCCINI. THEN
TAKE THE WALNUTS AND DRAIN THEM BUT
SAVE THE WATER IN CASE YOU NEED MORE
LIQUID FOR THE SAUCE AND THEN ADD
THE REST OF THE INGREDIENTS AND BLEND
INTO A SAUCE. THEN TAKE THE PESTO AND
TOSS THE ZUCCHINI WITH IT AND YOU
ARE DONE. YOU CAN ADD SLICED RED
PEPPERS IF YOU LIKE TO ADD MORE COLOR
AND NUTRITION. IT'S ALL UP TO YOU.

SPAGHETTI SQUASH WITH SPICY GARLIC SAUCE

1 WHOLE
SPAGHETTI
SQUASH
SLICED
CARROTS
SLICED GREEN
ZUCCHINI
1 CLOVE OF
GARLIC
$\frac{1}{2}$ CUP OF OLIVE OIL
$\frac{1}{2}$ TEASPOON OF RED CHILI PEPPERS
SALT AND PEPPER
THIS RECIPE IS SO EASY YOU WILL
WONDER WHY YOU DON'T EAT THIS
EVERYDAY! FIRST YOU PUT THE OLIVE OIL,
CHOPPED GARLIC, CHILI PEPPERS, AND SALT
AND PEPPER INTO A SMALL BOWL TO BLEND
THE FLAVORS. THEN YOU CUT THE SQUASH
IN HALF AND THEN START TO SCRAP THE
SQUASH OUT SO THAT THERE ARE STRINGS
OF THE SQUASH THAT LOOK LIKE
SPAGHETTI. I USE A SPOON WITH SHARP

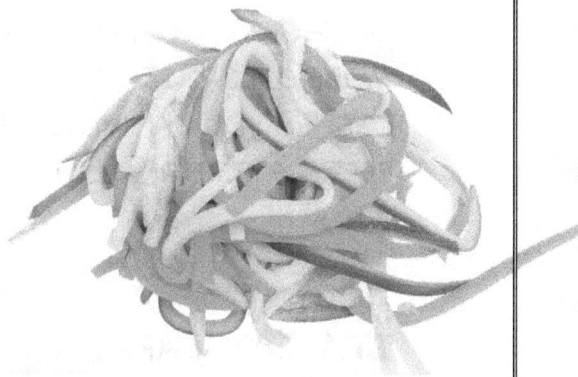

POINTS ON THE END SO THAT IT BREAKS
UP THE SQUASH BETTER. THEN YOU PUT
THE SQUASH IN A BOWL AND TOSS IT
WITH THE OLIVE OIL MIXTURE. IF YOU
WANT YOU CAN ADD SLIVERED RED PEPPERS
OR CHOPPED TOMATOES TO GIVE THE DISH
MORE COLOR. IF YOU DON'T LIKE HOT
DISHES YOU CAN ALSO OMIT THE CHILI
PEPPERS. IT'S REALLY UP TO YOUR TASTE
BUDS.

ITALIAN CAPRESE TOWERS

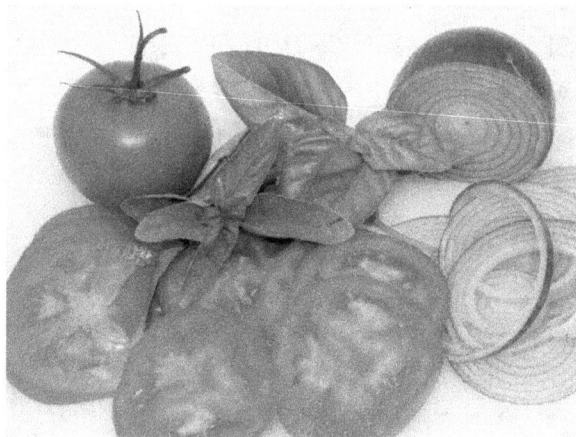

3-4 LARGE HEIRLOOM TOMATOES

SLICED ONION (WHICHEVER KIND YOU LIKE BEST)
2 CUPS SLICED MARINATED PORTOBELLO'S (IN A BOWL SOAK THE SLICED MUSHROOMS IN ½ CUP BALSAMIC VINEGAR, ½ CUP TAMARI, AND ¼ CUP OLIVE OIL FOR 4-6 HOURS)
PESTO FROM RECIPE NUMBER 9
RAW RICOTTA

FIRST SLICE THE TOMATOES. ON A LARGE PLATE ARRANGE THE INGREDIENTS IN LAYERS STARTING WITH THE TOMATOES, THEN PESTO, THEN PORTABELLAS, THEN RAW RICOTTA (WHICH IS 2 CUPS RAW PINE NUTS, SALT AND PEPPER, 3 TABLESPOONS OF LEMON JUICE, 1 TABLESPOON OF NUTRITIONAL YEAST, AND A COUPLE TEASPOONS OF OLIVE OIL. PLACE ALL INGREDIENTS IN A FOOD PROCESSOR UNTIL COMBINED WELL) AND FINALLY THE ONION. KEEP BUILDING LITTLE TOWERS ON THE LARGE PLATE SO THAT EVERYONE GETS ONE OR TWO.

LASAGNA

4-5 THINLY SLICED ZUCCHINI
3-4 CUPS MARINATED PORTOBELLO'S
(RECIPE 11)
RAW RICOTTA (IN RECIPE 11)
6-8 MEDIUM TOMATOES
1 CUP CHOPPED BASIL
1 CLOVE OF GARLIC
¼ CUP OLIVE OIL
1 TABLESPOON OREGANO OR ITALIAN
SPICES

FIRST START BY MAKING THE TOMATO
SAUCE. USING A VITAMIXER PUT THE
TOMATOES, BASIL, GARLIC, OLIVE OIL
SPICES, AND SALT AND PEPPER AND BLEND
UNTIL IT LOOKS LIKE A NICE THICK SAUCE.
NOW TAKE A GLASS BAKING DISH AND
START TO LAYER THE THINLY SLICED
ZUCCHINI, THEN RICOTTA SAUCE, TOMATO
SAUCE, AND THEN START ANOTHER LAYER
USING THE PORTABELLAS MUSHROOMS,
RICOTTA, AND THEN SAUCE. KEEP DOING
THIS UNTIL ALL OF THE INGREDIENTS ARE

USED UP AND TOP WITH SOME FRESHLY
CHOPPED BASIL.

STUFFED TOMATOES

7-8 LARGE TOMATOES
1 CUP CHOPPED BASIL
1 CLOVE GARLIC
1/8 CUP OF OLIVE OIL
SALT AND PEPPER
1 LARGE JICAMA PEELED
1 CUP RAW PINE NUTS SOAKED FOR 2
HOURS

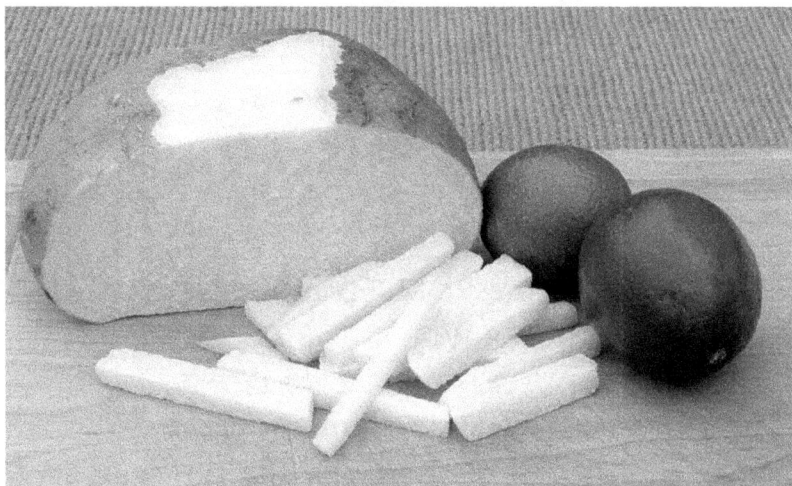

FIRST TAKE ALL OF THE TOMATOES AND
CUT INTO HALVES. THEN SCOOP OUT THE
INSIDE OF THE TOMATOES AND THEN
PLACE THEM IN A LARGE GLASS BAKING
SHEET. NEXT TAKE THE REST OF THE
INGREDIENTS AND BLEND IN A FOOD
PROCESSOR (LEAVING OUT $\frac{1}{2}$ CUP OF THE
BASIL FOR GARNISH) UNTIL SMOOTH AND
THEN FILL THE TOMATOES WITH THE
FILLING AND TOP WITH BASIL AND SERVE!

RAWVIOLI

1 EGGPLANT SLICED INTO VERY THIN
ROUNDS WITH A MANDOLIN
RAW RICOTTA (IN RECIPE 11)
PESTO SAUCE (RECIPE NUMBER 9)

PLACE THE THINLY SLICED EGGPLANT IN A
BOWL OF WATER WITH 1 TABLESPOON OF
SALT AND LET SOAK FOR 2 HOURS, THEN
DRAIN AND PAT DRY. NOW ADD THE RAW
RICOTTA AND FOLD IN HALF AND DRIZZLE

WITH OLIVE OIL AND PESTO SAUCE. YOU
CAN USE OTHER RAW SAUCES IF YOU
WOULD LIKE SUCH AS MARINARA, SUN
DRIED TOMATO, ETC.

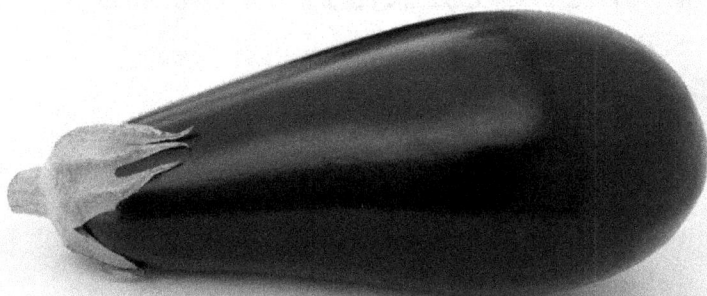

QUINOA SUMMER SALAD

1 CUP SPROUTED QUINOA (SOAK FOR 2
HOURS AND LET SPROUT FOR 1 DAY)
$\frac{1}{4}$ CUP CHOPPED MINT
1 CUP CUCUMBER DICED INTO SMALL PIECES
1 CUP RED AND GREEN PEPPERS CHOPPED
INTO SMALL PIECES

½ CUP CHOPPED PARSLEY
1 CLOVE OF GARLIC CHOPPED FINE
½ CUP OLIVE OIL
½ CUP LEMON JUICE
SALT AND PEPPER

MIX ALL INGREDIENTS IN A BOWL AND
SERVE.

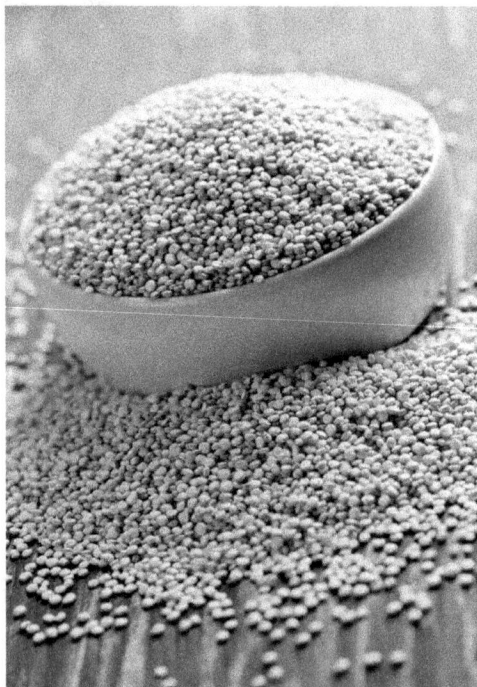

THAI WILD RICE SALAD

2 CUPS WILD RICE SOAKED FOR 9 HOURS
AND SPROUTED FOR 3-5 DAYS
1 CUP FINELY CHOPPED CELERY
1 CUP DICED CARROTS
½ CUP DICED RED PEPPER
1 TEASPOON OF GINGER
1 CLOVE OF GARLIC CHOPPED FINE
1 CUP CHOPPED RAW PEANUTS
1/2 CUP CHOPPED BASIL
1 TABLESPOON OF RAW ALMOND BUTTER
½ CUP CHOPPED CILANTRO
½-3/4 CUP LIME JUICE
¼ CUP OLIVE OIL
SALT AND PEPPER
DASH OF CHILI PEPPERS
MIX ALL INGREDIENTS TOGETHER AND
SERVE.

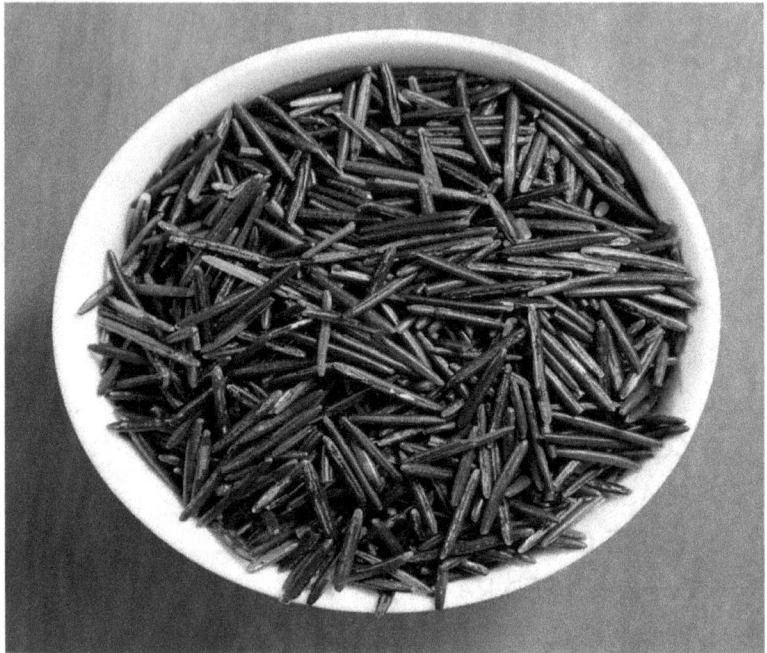

SWEET SUMMER WILD RICE SALAD

1   CUPS WILD RICE SOAKED FOR 9 HOURS AND
    SPROUTED FOR 3-5 DAYS

    1 LARGE RED APPLE CUT INTO SMALL PIECES

    1 CELERY STALK CUT INTO SMALL PIECES

    1 CUP OF DRIED CURRANTS

1 CUP CHOPPED RAW CASHEWS

¼ CUP CHOPPED PARSLEY

1 TABLESPOON OF OLIVE OIL

1 TEASPOON OF AGAVE NECTAR

SALT AND PEPPER

MIX ALL INGREDIENTS IN A BOWL AND SERVE.

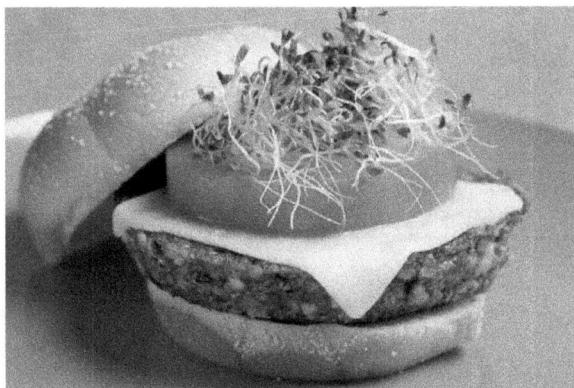

RAW BURGER

2   CUPS OF RAW WALNUTS

2   CUPS CARROTS
    ¼ CUP CELERY
1   CLOVE OF GARLIC

    1 SHALLOT

    1 TEASPOON OF AGAVE NECTAR

    1 PITTED DATE

    1 TABLESPOON OF OLIVE OIL

    1 TABLESPOON OF ITALIAN SEASONING

    SALT AND PEPPER

MIX ALL INGREDIENTS IN A FOOD
PROCESSOR UNTIL BLENDED. THE MIXTURE
SHOULD BE EASILY SHAPED INTO ROUND
PATTIES. THEN DRESS WITH SLICED
TOMATOES, ONIONS, CUCUMBERS, ETC.

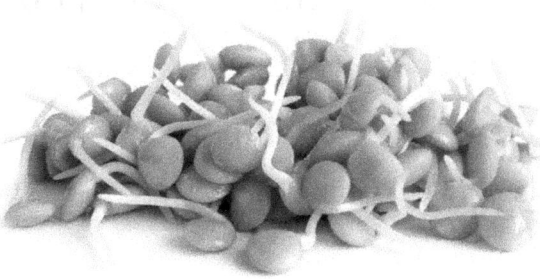

LENTIL SALAD

2 CUPS LENTILS SOAKED FOR 7 HOURS AND
SPROUTED FOR 3 DAYS

1/2 CUP LEMON JUICE

1 CUP CHOPPED PARSLEY

1 CUP SMALL DICED TOMATOES

$\frac{1}{4}$ CUP OLIVE OIL

SALT AND PEPPER

1 TEASPOON OF CUMIN

MIX ALL INGREDIENTS IN A BOWL AND
SERVE.

ITALIAN BARLEY SALAD

2 CUPS BARLEY SOAKED FOR 6 HOURS AND
SPROUTED FOR 2 DAYS

1 CUP SUNDRIED TOMATOES SOAKED FOR 4
HOURS

1 CLOVE OF GARLIC CHOPPED FINE

1 CUP PITTED AND CHOPPED BLACK OLIVES

$\frac{1}{2}$ CUP CHOPPED BASIL

$\frac{1}{4}$-1/2 CUP OLIVE OIL

SALT AND PEPPER

DRAIN THE SUN DRIED TOMATOES AND
CHOPPED INTO SMALL PIECES. TAKE THE
REST OF THE INGREDIENTS AND MIX IN A
BOWL AND SERVE.

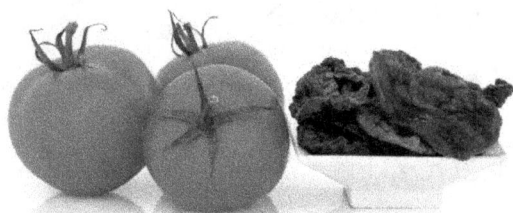

20 RAW DESSERTS

APPLE TARTLET

LEMON COOKIES

COCONUT HAYSTACKS

CHERRY CRISP

RAW KEY LIME PUDDING

ALMOND BUTTER BARS

APRICOT COOKIES

RAW PUMPKIN PIE

RAW MANGO PUDDING

RAW BANANA CREAM PIE

RAW CHOCOLATE CHIP COOKIES

RAW PECAN PIE

RAW CHOCOLATE CREAM PIE

RAW APPLE PIE

RAW CHEESECAKE

RAW BANANA CHOCOLATE ICE CREAM

RAW STRAWBERRY ICE CREAM

RAW RICE PUDDING

CHOCOLATE MACADAMIA PUDDING

OATMEAL COOKIES

APPLE TARTLETS WITH CACAO BANANA SAUCE

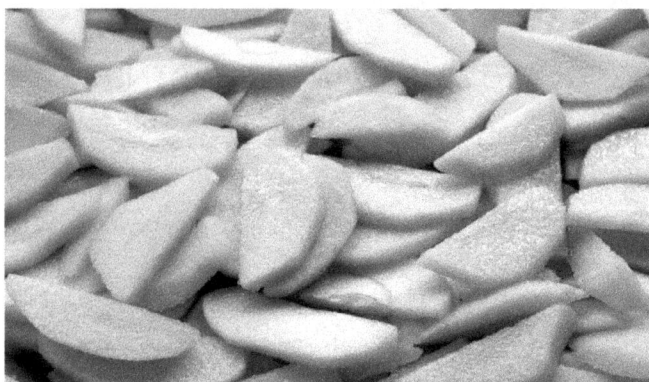

SERVES 4

CRUST:

3 CUPS YOUNG COCONUT, SHREDDED & DEHYDRATED
3 MEDJOOL DATES (PITTED)

BLEND COCONUT IN BLENDER OR FOOD PROCESSOR UNTIL FINE AND THEN ADD THE DATES AND BLEND. PRESS INTO 4, 3 INCH TARTLET PANS, LINED WITH PARCHMENT PAPER. FREEZE FOR 2 HOURS. TAKE OUT, DISCARD LINER, AND

LET STAND FOR 15 MINUTES BEFORE
ADDING FILLING.

FILLING:

4 CUPS APPLES, CORED & PEELED
½ CUP OF CHOPPED RAW ALMONDS
1 TSP CINNAMON
1/8 TSP NUTMEG
1/4 TSP FRESH GINGER
2 TBSP LEMON JUICE

PUT APPLES IN A FOOD PROCESSOR
UNTIL CHUNKY. STIR IN LEMON JUICE
AND SPICES. POUR INTO CRUST AND
TOP WITH CHOPPED ALMOND SAUCE.

CACAO BANANA SAUCE:

1 HALF OF BANANA
2 TSP OF RAW CACAO POWDER
1 YOUNG COCONUT
2 FRESH MEDJOOL
DATE

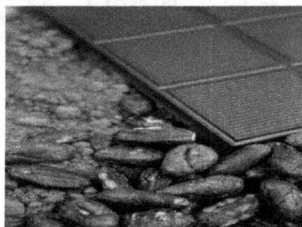

CAREFULLY OPEN UP
YOUNG COCONUTS
AND EMPTY LIQUID INTO A VITA MIXER

BLENDER. SCOOP OUT WHITE "MEAT"
OUT OF THE COCONUT AND PUT INTO
BLENDER AS WELL. ADD HALF OF THE
BANANA, PITTED DATES, AND COCOA
POWDER INTO BLENDER, BLEND UNTIL
SMOOTH.

PLACE TARTLET ON PLATE, SPOON
SAUCE ON TARTLET, AND SPRINKLE
CHOPPED ALMONDS ON TOP.

LEMON COOKIES

2 CUPS RAW CASHEWS (NOT SOAKED)
2 CUPS SHREDDED COCONUT
$\frac{1}{2}$ CUP LEMON JUICE
$\frac{1}{4}$ CUP OF ALMOND MILK
1/4 CUP LEMON ZEST
1/4 CUP MAPLE SYRUP

BLEND ALL INGREDIENTS IN A FOOD
PROCESSOR UNTIL SMOOTH AND THEN
FORM INTO COOKIE SHAPES AND
DEHYDRATE FOR 12HOURS AT 90
DEGREES.

COCONUT HAYSTACKS

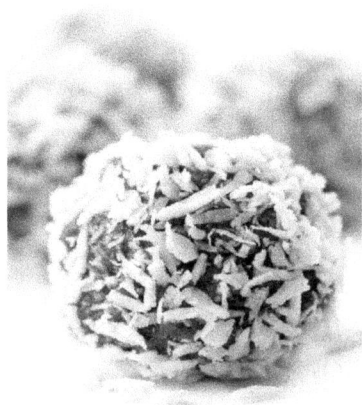

1 CUP COCONUT OIL
$\frac{1}{2}$ CUP RAW HONEY
$\frac{1}{4}$ CUP MAPLE SYRUP
$\frac{1}{2}$ CUP COCOA POWDER
1 TEASPOON VANILLA EXTRACT
4 CUPS SHREDDED COCONUT

BLEND ALL INGREDIENTS EXCEPT THE
SHREDDED COCONUT IN A FOOD
PROCESSOR UNTIL SMOOTH. NEXT ADD
THE COCONUT TO THE MIXTURE AND
FORM INTO ROUND BALLS AND PLACE
ON PARCHMENT PAPER AND FREEZE.

THEY WILL BECOME SOFT IF LEFT OUT
OF THE FREEZER FOR VERY LONG SO
BRING THEM OUT AROUND 15 MINUTES
BEFORE SERVING.

CHERRY CRISP

YIELD: 1 (8-INCH) CRISP

CRUMBLE TOPPING:
2 CUPS RAW WALNUTS OR PECANS
CHOPPED
½ CUP RAW OATS
1/2 CUP UNSWEETENED SHREDDED
DRIED COCONUT
1/4 TEASPOON GROUND CINNAMON
1/4 TEASPOON GROUND NUTMEG
1/4 TEASPOON SALT
1/2 CUP DRIED CHERRIES CHOPPED
8 PITTED MEDJOOL DATES GROUND UP
SMALL
1/4 CUP MAPLE SYRUP

FILLING:
30 OZ OF FROZEN CHERRIES FROZEN

THAWED AND DRAINED
3/4CUP PITTED MEDJOOL DATES,
SOAKED
1 TABLESPOON FRESH LEMON JUICE

BLEND ALL OF THE FILLING AND PUT
INTO A GLASS BAKING CONTAINER.
THEN TAKE THE CRUMBLE TOPPING AND
MIX BY HAND UNTIL SMOOTH AND
THEN PUT THE CRUMBLE ON TOP OF THE
CHERRIES.

RAW KEY LIME PUDDING

1 CUP YOUNG COCONUT MEAT
2 TABLESPOONS COCONUT BUTTER
$\frac{1}{2}$ CUP MACADAMIA NUTS
$\frac{1}{4}$ CUP COCONUT WATER
4 TABLESPOONS KEY LIME JUICE
1 KEY LIME FOR ZESTING
$\frac{1}{4}$ TEASPOON CELTIC SEA SALT
1 TABLESPOON OF MAPLE SYRUP

MIX THE MACADAMIA NUTS, WATER, COCONUT WATER AND LIME JUICE IN A HIGH-POWERED BLENDER, VITA MIXER, OR FOOD PROCESSOR AND BLEND UNTIL SMOOTH. THEN ADD ALL OTHER INGREDIENTS AND BLEND UNTIL SMOOTH. REFRIGERATE FOR AT LEAST 1 HOUR BEFORE SERVING SO THAT PUDDING MAY THICKEN. THEN TOP WITH KEY LIME ZEST.

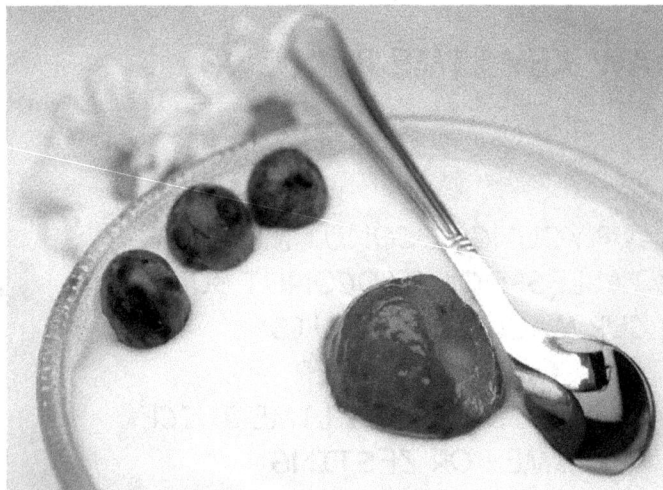

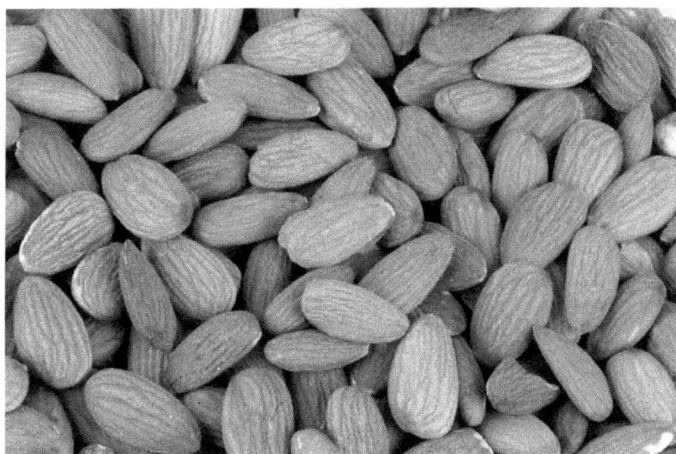

ALMOND BUTTER BARS

3/4 CUP RAW ALMOND BUTTER
1/4 CUP MACADAMIA NUT BUTTER
1/2 CUP RAW HONEY
1 CUP RAW SESAME SEEDS
1/4 CUP OF RAW CACAO POWDER
1/2 CUP OF SHREDDED COCONUT

MIX ALL INGREDIENTS IN A FOOD
PROCESSOR ON SLOW AND THEN
REMOVE AND PUT INTO A GLASS PAN
AND THEN TOP WITH CHOPPED RAW
ALMONDS!

APRICOT COOKIES

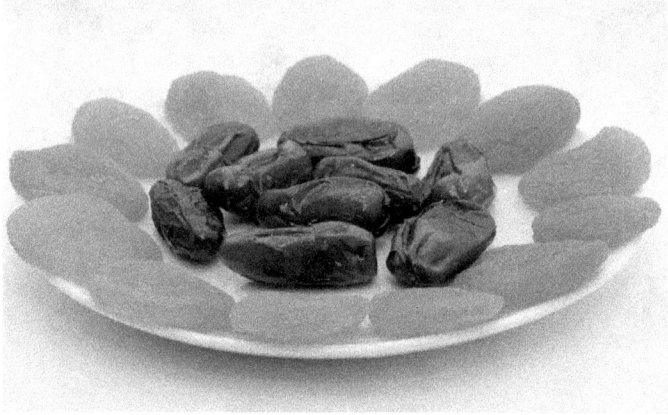

2 CUPS OATS SOAKED
2 CUPS DRIED APRICOTS
1 CUP OF DATES PITTED
½ CUP DRIED FIGS SOAKED
1 CUP FINELY GROUND FLAXSEEDS
1 CUP PECANS CHOPPED
½ CUP MAPLE SYRUP
(SAVE THE WATER FROM SOAKING THE
FIGS)

IN A VITA MIXER ADD THE OATS,
DATES, DRIED FIGS; SOAK WATER,
FINELY GROUND FLAXSEEDS, AND
MAPLE SYRUP. TAKE THE MIXTURE AND

ADD THE CHOPPED APRICOTS AND
CHOPPED PECANS AND FORM INTO
COOKIES AND DEHYDRATE FOR 100
DEGREES FOR 4 HOURS ON EACH SIDE.

RAW PUMPKIN PIE

CRUST:
1 CUP RAW PECANS GROUND UP FINE
1 TBSP. LEMON ZEST
6 DATES PITTED
MIX ALL INGREDIENTS IN A FOOD
PROCESSOR UNTIL SMOOTH AND THEN
SPREAD OUT EVENLY IN DISH.

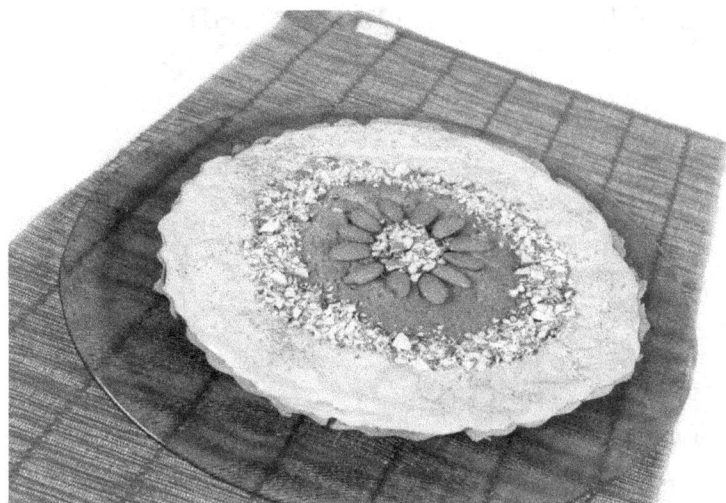

FILLING

2 CUPS RAW PUMPKIN CUT UP
1 AVOCADO PITTED
1 TBSP LEMON JUICE
2 TEASPOONS OF PUMPKIN SPICES
2 TABLESPOONS OF MAPLE SYRUP
2 TABLESPOON OF FINELY GROUND
FLAXSEEDS
1/2 TEASPOON FRESH GINGER

PUT ALL INGREDIENTS IN FOOD
PROCESSOR AND PROCESS UNTIL
SMOOTH. PUT INTO DISH ONTO CRUST
AND SPREAD EVENLY. SET IN
FRIDGE TO ALLOW TO SET SOME MORE.
SERVE WITH FOLLOWING WHIP.

WHIP:

1 CUP OF MACADAMIA NUTS
7 PITTED DATES
1 TBSP. LEMON JUICE
2-3 TABLESPOONS OF ORANGE JUICE

PUT ALL INGREDIENTS IN BLENDER AND
LET PROCESS UNTIL SMOOTH. KEEP
ADDING THE ORANGE JUICE TO KEEP

THE MIXTURE THIN ENOUGH TO WHIP
IN THE BLENDER.

YOU WANT THE WHIP TO BE SMOOTH
AND THICK BUT LOOSE ENOUGH TO
JUST ABOUT POUR.

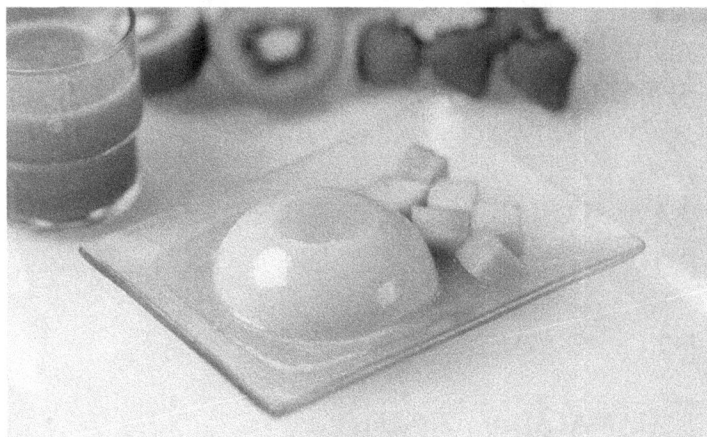

RAW MANGO PUDDING

2 MANGOS
1 CUP OF MACADAMIA NUTS SOAKED
FOR 4 HOURS
1 CUP YOUNG COCONUT MEAT
1/8 CUP OF LIME JUICE

SHREDDED COCONUT & CHOPPED
MACADAMIA NUTS FOR THE TOPPING.

USE A VEGETABLE PEELER TO PEEL
MANGOS. THEN CUT THE MANGO INTO
PIECES THROWING AWAY THE PIT.
DRAIN THE MACADAMIA NUTS AND PUT
ALL THE INGREDIENTS IN A BLENDER
AND BLEND UNTIL SMOOTH. THEN ADD
SHREDDED COCONUT AND CHOPPED
MACADAMIA TO TASTE.

RAW BANANA COCONUT CREAM PIE

FOR THE CRUST:

1 CUP MACADAMIA NUTS
½ CUP SHREDDED DRY COCONUT
1 TSP COCONUT OIL
2 TABLESPOONS OF RAW HONEY
PINCH OF SALT

FOR THE FILLING:

2 CUPS YOUNG COCONUT MEAT ABOUT 2 YOUNG
COCONUTS
½ CUP RAW COCONUT OIL

3 TABLESPOONS OF RAW HONEY
2 TABLESPOON LIME JUICE
$\frac{1}{4}$ TEASPOON SALT
$\frac{1}{2}$ TEASPOON VANILLA EXTRACT
3 BANANAS (2 OF THEM SLICED)

PREPARING THE CRUST
BLEND FIRST 5 INGREDIENTS IN A FOOD PROCESSOR THEN ADD MORE HONEY IF NEEDED TO MAKE CRUST STICKY. LINE PIE PAN WITH SARAN WRAP AND PRESS CRUST ON TOP. PLACE IN FREEZER WHILE MAKING THE FILLING.

PREPARING THE FILLING

BLEND THE REST OF THE INGREDIENTS, (**EXCEPT BANANAS THAT ARE SLICED**) IN A VITA MIXER UNTIL SMOOTH.
MAKE SURE THERE IS ENOUGH LIQUID TO HAVE THE INGREDIENTS MOVING, YOU MAY NEED TO ADD COCONUT WATER. TAKE CRUST OUT FROM FREEZER AND PLACE SLICED BANANAS ON TOP OF CRUST. POUR FILLING ON

TOP OF BANANAS. PLACE IN FREEZER
FOR 3-4 HOURS TO SET.
TOP WITH SHREDDED COCONUT! YUM!

RAW "CHOCOLATE CHIP" COOKIES

1 CUP RAW WALNUTS
1 CUP PECANS
1 CUP MACADAMIA NUTS
15 DATES
1 TEASPOON OF CINNAMON
½ TSP SALT
2 TABLESPOON RAW COCONUT OIL
4 TABLESPOONS CACAO NIBS

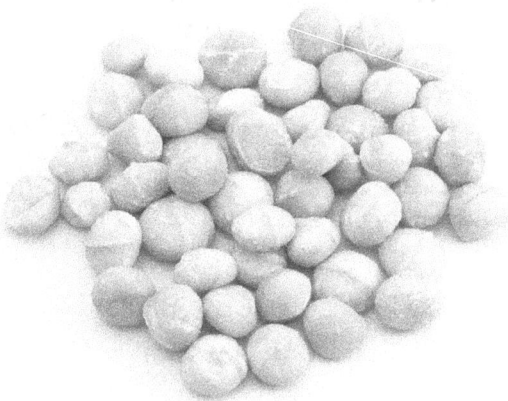

PLACE DATES IN FOOD PROCESSOR AND MIX UNTIL SMOOTH. ADD NUTS, CINNAMON, SALT AND COCONUT OIL AND MIX IT ALL UP, AGAIN UNTIL SMOOTH. ONCE SMOOTH, ADD CACAO NIBS AND BLEND JUST UNTIL NIBS ARE WELL DISTRIBUTED. AFTER INGREDIENTS ARE MIXED, REMOVE FROM FOOD PROCESSOR AND USE A SPOON TO MAKE FLAT COOKIE SHAPES. REFRIGERATE BEFORE EATING.

RAW PECAN PIE

FOR THE CRUST:

1 CUP MACADAMIA NUTS
½ CUP SHREDDED DRY COCONUT
1 TSP COCONUT OIL
2 TABLESPOONS OF RAW HONEY
PINCH OF SALT

FOR THE FILLING:

3 CUPS PECANS PROCESSED IN A FOOD
PROCESSOR UNTIL SMOOTH
30 PITTED DATES
2 CUPS SHREDDED, DRIED COCONUT
1/2 TEASPOON SALT
1 TEASPOON CINNAMON
1/2 CUP PECANS, CHOPPED

PREPARING THE CRUST

BLEND FIRST 5 INGREDIENTS IN A
FOOD PROCESSOR THEN ADD
MORE HONEY IF NEEDED TO MAKE
CRUST STICKY. LINE PIE PAN
WITH SARAN WRAP AND PRESS
CRUST ON TOP. PLACE IN FREEZER
WHILE MAKING THE FILLING.

FOR THE FILLING:

IN FOOD PROCESSOR, PROCESS DATES
UNTIL SMOOTH (OR AS CLOSE TO
SMOOTH AS YOU CAN GET). ADD THE
SMOOTH PECANS, COCONUT, SALT, AND
CINNAMON. PROCESS UNTIL
EVERYTHING IS WELL MIXED. REMOVE

FROM FOOD PROCESSOR AND THEN
PLACE INGREDIENTS IN THE PREPARED
CRUST. TOP WITH THE EXTRA CHOPPED
PECANS AND THEN REFRIGERATE FOR 1-
2 HOURS.

RAW CHOCOLATE CREAM PIE

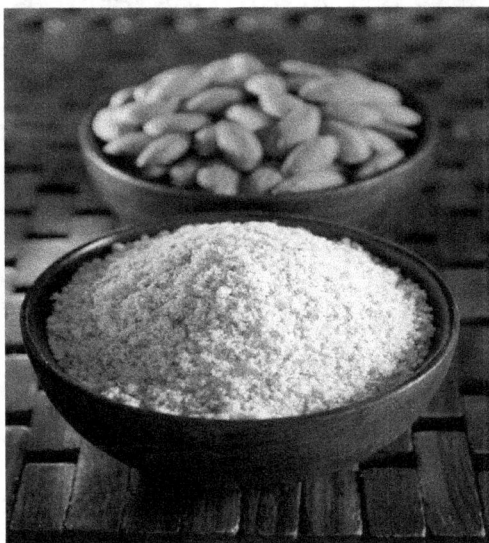

CRUST
1/2 CUP ALMONDS
1/2 CUP PECANS
1/2 CUP OF BRAZIL NUTS
 8 PITTED DATES

1/4 CUP AGAVE SYRUP
1/4 CUP CACAO POWDER
PINCH SEA SALT

PUT NUTS INTO FOOD PROCESSOR AND
PROCESS UNTIL GROUND.
PLACE THE REST OF THE INGREDIENTS
IN PROCESSOR WITH NUTS AND
PROCESS UNTIL COMBINED. SPREAD
ONTO A PIE PAN USING YOUR HANDS.

CREAM FILLING
MEAT OF 2 YOUNG THAI COCONUTS
2 AVOCADO
6 PITTED DATES
1/2 CUP CACAO POWDER
2 TABLESPOONS OF MAPLE SYRUP

PLACE ALL INGREDIENTS IN FOOD
PROCESSOR AND PROCESS UNTIL WELL
COMBINED. IF FILLING IS NOT SWEET
OR CHOCOLATY ENOUGH FOR YOU ADD A
MORE SYRUP OR MORE CACAO POWDER
RESPECTIVELY. SPREAD INTO INSIDE OF
PIE CRUST. TOP WITH SOME SLICED
STRAWBERRIES OR RASPBERRIES FOR
ADDED FLAVOR.

CHILL IN REFRIGERATOR FOR 1-2 HOURS
AND SERVE.

RAW APPLE PIE

CRUST:

1 ½ CUPS OF RAW ALMONDS SOAKED FOR
4-6 HOURS
1/8 CUP OF OLIVE OIL
1 TABLESPOON OF COCONUT OIL
PINCH OF SALT

FILLING:

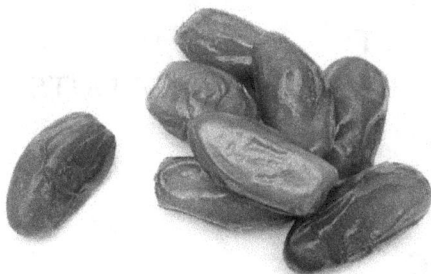

4-5 RED APPLES CORED
5 PITTED DATES
1 TEASPOON OF COCONUT OIL
2 TABLESPOONS OF MAPLE SYRUP
1 TEASPOON OF CINNAMON

PINCH OF SALT

BLEND THE ALMONDS IN A FOOD
PROCESSOR AND THEN ADD THE REST
OF THE CRUST INGREDIENTS. PUT THE
CRUST INTO A GLASS PIE PAN. NEXT
TAKE THE FILLING INGREDIENTS AND
BLEND TOGETHER AND POUR INTO THE
CRUST PAN. CHILL IN THE
REFRIGERATOR FOR 1-2 HOURS.

RAW CHEESECAKE

THE CRUST:
2 CUPS RAW MACADAMIA NUTS
8 PITTED DATES
$\frac{1}{4}$ CUP DRIED COCONUT

FILLING:

3 CUPS CASHEWS SOAKED FOR AT
LEAST 3 HOURS
$\frac{3}{4}$ CUP LEMON JUICE
$\frac{3}{4}$ CUPS MAPLE SYRUP
$\frac{3}{4}$ CUP COCONUT OIL

MEAT FROM ONE RAW YOUNG COCONUT
½ CUP COCOA NIBS

MAKE THE CRUST BY PROCESSING THE
INGREDIENTS IN A FOOD PROCESSOR.
PRESS THE INGREDIENTS INTO A
SPRING FORM PAN. NEXT BLEND THE
CASHEWS, LEMON, MAPLE SYRUP,
COCONUT OIL, YOUNG COCONUT MEAT,
VANILLA, AND SEA SALT. BLEND UNTIL
SMOOTH. POUR THE MIXTURE ONTO
THE CRUST AND TOP WITH COCOA NIBS
AND THEN FREEZE UNTIL FIRM.

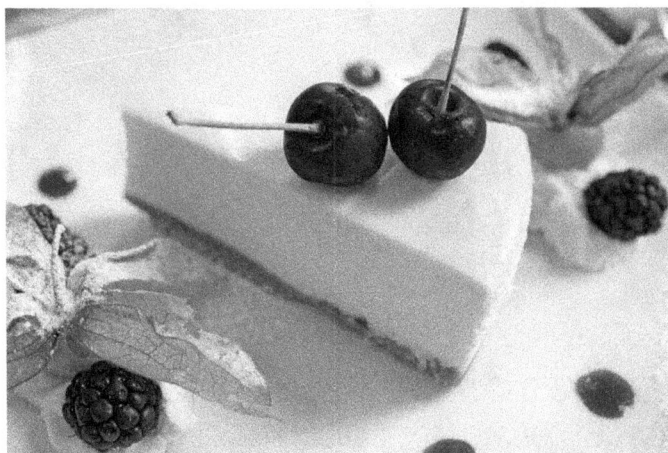

RAW BANANA & CHOCOLATE ICE CREAM

3 BANANAS SLICED AND THEN FROZEN
$\frac{1}{4}$ C RAW CACAO OR COCOA POWDER
2 T RAW HONEY
1 TEASPOON VANILLA
1 PINCH OF SALT
$\frac{1}{4}$ CUP COCOA NIBS

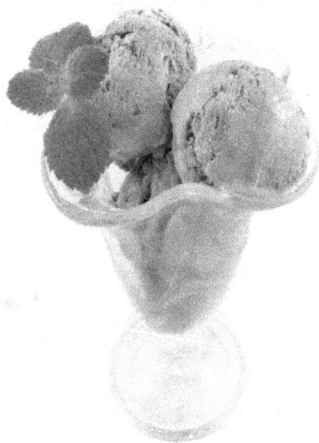

REMOVE BANANAS FROM FREEZER AND
PLACE THEM IN A FOOD PROCESSOR;
ADD CACAO, HONEY, SALT AND VANILLA
AND MIX UNTIL THICK AND CREAMY.

ADD COCOA NIBS AND BLEND QUICKLY, JUST UNTIL THEY ARE MIXED THROUGH, BUT NOT GROUND TOO SMALL. POUR MIXTURE INTO A LOAF PAN AND COVER WITH SARAN WRAP. PLACE IN FREEZER. WHEN SERVING, REMOVE FROM FREEZER 5 MINUTES BEFORE. SCOOP AND SERVE, JUST AS YOU WOULD REGULAR ICE CREAM.

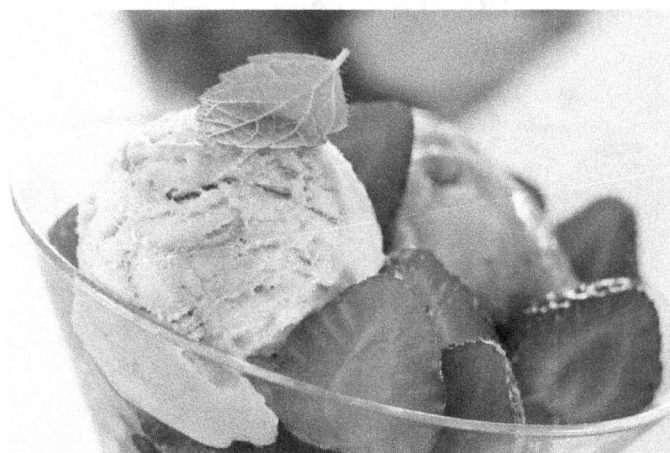

RAWBERRY ICE CREAM

1 FROZEN BANANA
1 CUP FRESH STRAWBERRIES
$\frac{1}{4}$ CUP RAW HONEY

THE MEAT FROM ONE RAW COCONUT
2 CUPS RAW CASHEWS
PINCH OF SALT

BLEND ALL INGREDIENTS IN A FOOD
PROCESSOR UNTIL SMOOTH AND THEN
PLACE IN A CONTAINER AND FREEZE.

RAW RICE PUDDING

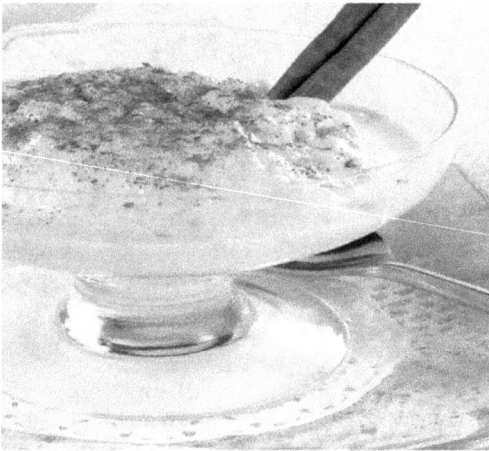

1 $\frac{1}{2}$ CUP OF BROWN RICE SOAKED FOR 3
DAYS
4 YOUNG COCONUTS

2 TEASPOONS OF CINNAMON
1 TEASPOON OF NUTMEG
1 TEASPOON OF VANILLA
2 TABLESPOONS OF MAPLE SYRUP

IN A VITA MIXER BLEND THE COCONUT MEAT AND ONLY 2 CUPS OF THE COCONUT WATER, CINNAMON, VANILLA, AND MAPLE SYRUP. BLEND UNTIL SMOOTH. IN A LARGE BOWL MIX IN THE RICE AND THE BLENDED INGREDIENTS AND LET SET IN THE REFRIGERATOR FOR 1 HOUR.

CHOCOLATE MACADAMIA PUDDING

2 CUPS RAW MACADAMIA NUTS
2 CUPS PITTED DATES
½ CUP COCOA POWDER
1 CUP OF COCONUT WATER

BLEND ALL INGREDIENTS TOGETHER
UNTIL SMOOTH AND SERVE.

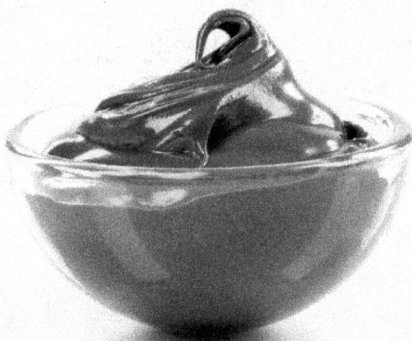

RAW OATMEAL COOKIES

2 CUPS OATS SOAKED OVERNIGHT
1/2 CUP OF ALMOND MILK
10 PITTED DATES
1 CUP OF RAW ALMONDS

$\frac{1}{2}$ CUP RAISONS
$\frac{1}{2}$ CUP MAPLE SYRUP

MIX ALL INGREDIENTS IN A FOOD
PROCESSOR (EXCEPT THE RAISONS) AND
BLEND. NEXT ADD THE RAISONS. NOW
TAKE SMALL AMOUNTS OF THE DOUGH
AND FLATTEN ON A DEHYDRATOR
SHEETS SO THEY RESEMBLE COOKIES
AND DEHYDRATE FOR 12 HOURS AT 110
DEGREES. YUM!

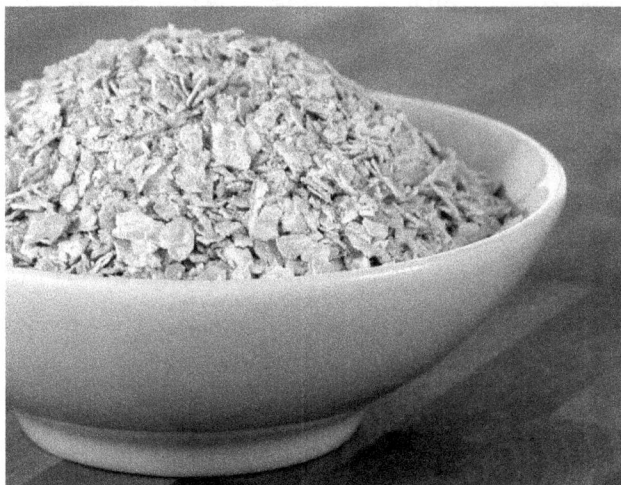

THANKS FOR TAKING THE TIME TO TRY THESE HEALTHY RECIPES. YOU WILL BE GLAD YOU DID. ALSO I WOULD LIKE TO TAKE A MINUTE TO TELL YOU HOW IMPORTANT IT IS TO PURCHASE ORGANIC PRODUCE.

WHY EAT ORGANIC?

EATING ORGANIC IS A CHOICE THAT MOST OF US PONDER EVERY DAY. I KNOW I ALWAYS CHOSE ORGANIC WHEN I CAN OR WHEN I HAVE ENOUGH MONEY. BUT WHAT DOES ORGANIC MEAN? THE FIRST ORGANIC PRODUCE LAW WAS IN 1990 FROM CONGRESS AND IT STATED THAT FOOD GROWN WITHOUT PESTICIDES, FUNGICIDES, OR NOT GENETICALLY MODIFIED WOULD BE CONSIDERED ORGANIC. PESTICIDES ARE TOXIC AND BAD FOR THE ENVIRONMENT, FARMERS, AND FOR YOU AND YOUR FAMILY. GENETICALLY MODIFIED FOOD (FOOD THAT IS MADE TO BE LARGER, BETTER COLORING, AND PEST RESISTANT) HAS BEEN QUESTIONED BY MANY PEOPLE. NO ONE REALLY KNOWS THE

LONG -TERM EFFECTS OF THIS ON YOUR
BODY.

SOME OF THE HIGHEST LEVELS OF
PESTICIDE RESIDUE ON PRODUCE THAT IS
CONSIDERED NOT ORGANIC ARE APRICOTS,
NECTARINES, GREEN BEANS, POTATOES,
BANANAS, CUCUMBERS, CELERY, CORN,
PEPPERS, CHERRIES, APPLES, SPINACH,
TOMATOES, SOY BEANS, RICE,
STRAWBERRIES, DATES, CARROTS, GRAPES,
PEACHES, PEARS, LEMONS, MILK, AND
SWEET POTATOES. SO I GUESS IF YOU
DON'T EAT ANY OF THESE YOUR O.K. WELL
THAT SOUNDS LIKE A LOT OF FRUITS AND
VEGETABLES TO ME. THERE HAVE BEEN
NUMEROUS STUDIES SHOWING HOW
FOODS GROWN WITHOUT PESTICIDES AND
FUNGICIDES HAVE MORE NUTRITIONAL
VALUE AND A MUCH HIGHER MINERAL
CONTENT. EVEN IF THE NUTRITIONAL
LEVEL WAS A LITTLE BETTER DON'T YOU
THINK THAT YOU WOULD WANT THAT FOR
YOU AND YOUR FAMILY? IT IS ALSO VERY
IMPORTANT TO DRINK ORGANIC MILK OR
MILK PRODUCTS THAT HAVE BEEN MADE
WITHOUT GROWTH HORMONE AND

ANTIBIOTICS. I THINK I WILL TAKE MY
ANTIBIOTICS FROM THE DOCTOR THANK
YOU!

SOME WAYS TO GET MORE ORGANIC
PRODUCE IN YOUR DAILY DIET IS TO SHOP
AT LOCAL FARMERS MARKETS, ASK YOUR
LOCAL SUPERMARKET TO CARRY MORE
ORGANIC CHOICES, AT THE SEASONAL
FARMERS MARKETS BUY EXTRA SO YOU CAN
DEHYDRATE OR FREEZE YOUR EXTRAS FOR
THE WINTER MONTHS, START A GARDEN,
ORDER ONLINE AND HAVE IT DELIVERED,
BECOME A MEMBER OF A FOOD CO-OP,
START A FOOD CO-OP, OR PARTICIPATE IN A
ORGANIC FOOD BUYING CLUB. THESE ARE
SOME SIMPLE WAYS TO INTRODUCE
ORGANIC FOOD INTO YOU AND YOUR
FAMILY'S DIET. YOU AND YOUR FAMILY ARE
WORTH IT. THE MORE DEMAND IN THE
MARKET PLACE FOR ORGANIC PRODUCE THE
SOY BEANS, RICE, STRAWBERRIES, DATES,
CARROTS, GRAPES, PEACHES, PEARS,
LEMONS, MILK, AND SWEET POTATOES. SO
I GUESS IF YOU DON'T EAT ANY OF THESE
YOUR O.K. WELL THAT SOUNDS LIKE A LOT
OF FRUITS AND VEGETABLES TO ME. THERE

HAVE BEEN NUMEROUS STUDIES SHOWING HOW FOODS GROWN WITHOUT PESTICIDES AND FUNGICIDES HAVE MORE NUTRITIONAL VALUE AND A MUCH HIGHER MINERAL CONTENT. EVEN IF THE NUTRITIONAL LEVEL WAS A LITTLE BETTER DON'T YOU THINK THAT YOU WOULD WANT THAT FOR YOU AND YOUR FAMILY? IT IS ALSO VERY IMPORTANT TO DRINK ORGANIC MILK OR MILK PRODUCTS THAT HAVE BEEN MADE WITHOUT GROWTH HORMONE AND ANTIBIOTICS. I THINK I WILL TAKE MY ANTIBIOTICS FROM THE DOCTOR THANK YOU!

SOME WAYS TO GET MORE ORGANIC PRODUCE IN YOUR DAILY DIET IS TO SHOP AT LOCAL FARMERS MARKETS, ASK YOUR LOCAL SUPERMARKET TO CARRY MORE ORGANIC CHOICES, AT THE SEASONAL FARMERS MARKETS BUY EXTRA SO YOU CAN DEHYDRATE OR FREEZE YOUR EXTRAS FOR THE WINTER MONTHS, START A GARDEN, ORDER ONLINE AND HAVE IT DELIVERED, BECOME A MEMBER OF A FOOD CO-OP, START A FOOD CO-OP, OR PARTICIPATE IN A ORGANIC FOOD BUYING CLUB. THESE ARE

SOME SIMPLE WAYS TO INTRODUCE
ORGANIC FOOD INTO YOU AND YOUR
FAMILY'S DIET. YOU AND YOUR FAMILY ARE
WORTH IT. THE MORE DEMAND IN THE
MARKET PLACE FOR ORGANIC PRODUCE THE
CHEAPER IT WILL EVENTUALLY BE. DO YOUR
PART IN HELPING THE ENVIRONMENT AND
SUPPORT YOUR LOCAL FARMERS. IT ONLY
TAKES A FEW PEOPLE IN EVERY TOWN TO
MAKE A DIFFERENCE. LET IT BE YOU!

ABOUT THE AUTHOR:

B.S. Science in Physical Anthropology minor in business, and Culinary Arts Degree.

Advocate for organic, vegetarian, vegan, raw food diets, writing, yoga, swimming, biking, and running 5 K's!. I have been a vegetarian/vegan/raw foodist for over 20 years. I have also worked in real estate for over ten years and have several websites to help people who are interested in raw food http://www.Recipes4RawFood.com and http://www.RawFoodForToday.com .

I have also started the Raw Foods Association with my husband so that others can become members of a larger healthy group and its website is www.RawFoodsAssociation.com!

For more information on how to order books, original articles, become a member of the Raw Foods Association, and updates on future projects go to www.recipes4rawfood.com, www.rawfoodfortoday.com, and www.rawfoodsassociation.com.

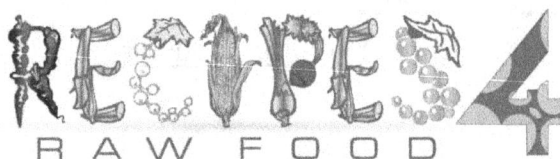

RECIPES 4
RAW FOOD

1314 E Las Olas Blvd

Fort Lauderdale, FL 33301

Recipes4RawFood@yahoo.com

I HOPE YOU ENJOY MY RAW RECIPES!
YOU SHOULD CHECK OUT MORE OF MY
RECIPES AT
WWW.RECIPES4RAWFOOD.COM AND
WWW.RAWFOODFORTODAY.COM

IF YOU HAVE ANY SUGGESTIONS,
COMMENTS, OR CORRECTIONS PLEASE
FEEL FREE TO EMAIL ME AT
RECIPES4RAWFOOD@YAHOO.COM.

Index

A

B

C

N

Nectarine Page 53
Nori 92-94
Nuts Page 27

O

Oats Page 122, 126, 144
Orange Page 40-44, 48, 51, 52, 58, 78, 79, 92, 128

P

Papaya Page 47, 92
Pasta Page 99
Peas Page 65
Peach Page 42, 147
Peanut Page 75, 79, 91
Pear Page 52, 147
Pecans Page 29, 122, 126, 127, 131, 133-135
Pesto Page 89, 96, 100, 104, 107, 108
Pies Page 18, 127, 130, 133, 135, 137
Pine Nuts Page 95, 106
Pizza Page 95, 96
Pudding Page 124, 129, 142, 143
Pumpkin Page 127

V

Vegan Page 30, 32

W

Walnut Page 29, 31, 97, 101, 112, 122, 131
Wraps Page 89, 90, 92, 93, 98
Watermelon Page 68, 77, 78

Y

Z

Zucchini Page 59, 81, 93, 99-102, 105

www.ingramcontent.com/pod-product-compliance
Lightning Source LLC
Chambersburg PA
CBHW060859280326
41934CB00007B/1110